Sexual

Health:

A

Nurse's

Guide

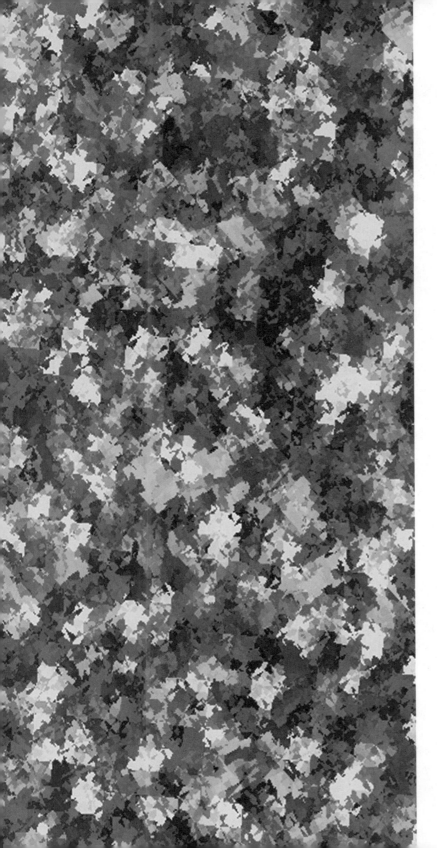

Sexual Health: A Nurse's Guide

Carole Israeloff Zawid

PhD, RNCS, OCN

Marriage and Family Therapist

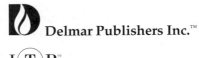

Delmar Publishers Inc.™

I T P™

NOTICE TO THE READER

Cover Design: J² Designs

Delmar Publishing Team
Publisher: David C. Gordon
Senior Acquisitions Editor: Bill Burgower
Assistant Editor: Debra M. Flis
Project Editor: Danya M. Plotsky
Production Coordinator: Barbara A. Bullock
Art and Design Coordinators: Megan K. DeSantis
                              Timothy J. Conners

For information, address

Delmar Publishers Inc.
3 Columbia Circle, Box 15015,
Albany, NY 12212-5015

Printed in the United States of America
Published simultaneously in Canada
by Nelson Canada,
a division of The Thomson Corporation

1 2 3 4 5 6 7 8 9 10 XXX 00 99 98 97 96 95 94

Library of Congress Cataloging-in-Publication Data

Zawid, Carole S.
    Sexual health: a nurse's guide / Carole S. Zawid.
        p. cm — (RealNursing series)
    Includes bibliographical references and index.
    ISBN 0-8273-5685-4
    1 Hygene, Sexual. 2. Nursing. 3. Sex. I. Title. II. Series. [DNLM: 1. Sex behavior—nurses' instruction. 2. Nurse-Patient Relations. WY 87 Z395 1994]
RA778.Z39
613.9'5—dc20
DNLM/DLC
for Library of Congress   93-34696
                                                                    CIP

REALNURSING SERIES
Alice M. Stein, MA, RN, Series Editor
Medical College of Pennsylvania

Dedication

This book is dedicated to three very special groups of people. First, it is dedicated to all of the patients that may benefit from this knowledge. It is also dedicated to all of the nurses who will take the time and energy to read this book and therefore become the catalyst toward their patients' positive entitlement of having healthy and pleasurable sexual functioning. Finally, it is dedicated to my husband Joe, and my four children, Jennifer, Steven, Brian, and Eric, who all helped me in their own unique and special way so that I could have the privilege of writing this book.

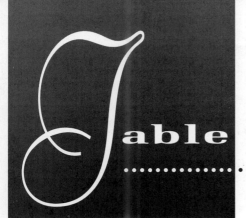

Table of Contents

PART III
MEDICAL ISSUES AND SEXUALITY

PART IV
SEXUAL PROBLEMS AND POSITIVE INTERVENTIONS

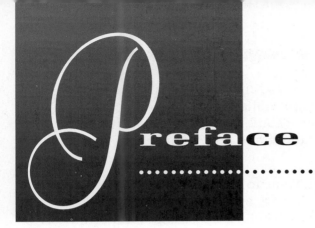

reface

Sexuality begins in utero and typically extends to the last moments of life. However, throughout the life span, health problems can and often do affect sexual expression and intimacy. Unfortunately, as the role of the nurse becomes increasingly complex and technologically more narrowly focused, issues related to sexual concerns are frequently not addressed either in nursing schools or in the health institutions in which nurses are employed. Compounding this problem is a culture that addresses sexual concerns only with a great amount of unease and discomfort. Unfortunately, since nurses' knowledge of sexual issues is often superficial, "normal" sexual concerns are frequently not discussed with patients. This is a tragedy, not only for patients but also for nurses, because sexuality is an inherent part of our beings, and it certainly does not become less important as patients enter the health care system.

This book is written in response to this dilemma. It is an attempt to give nurses the cognitive and affective resources they need to adequately address their patients' concerns. In an era when sex education is at best "spotty" the void must be filled with appropriate information. Sexual expression does not exist in a vacuum; it is always a reflection of the culture. If that culture not only distrusts sexual expression but is also extremely uncomfortable discussing issues that are intrinsically important to our emotional and physical health then professionals such as nurses are needed to help patients deal with health issues as they relate to sexuality.

This book is based on the philosophy that sexuality is an important experience throughout the life cycle, and also that certain issues are more relevant in specific periods of that cycle. Chapters 1 and 2 discuss the meaning of sexuality and give a historical overview of our attitudes toward sexuality. Chapters 3 through 7 discuss sexuality through the context of the total life cycle—from *in utero* through old age—and focus on current topics relevant to these ages. Chapters 8 through 13 describe the impact of disease on sexuality and offer specific interventions that the nurse can use to help patients and their significant others cope with these challenges. Finally, chapters 14 through 16 present many of the techniques necessary to enable the nurse to do a sexual history and begin to understand and recognize the concepts of sex therapy.

As you read this book you will come to recognize that the expression of sexuality is based on a multiplicity of influences. These include culture, gender, race, age, religion, and life experiences. Unfortunately, it is beyond the scope of this book to acknowledge the total range and effect of all of these diverse factors.

Therefore, the book is based on broad generalizations regarding sexual expression in our culture. However, it is the hope of the author that these generalizations will be viewed as the foundation toward enabling your patients toward positive sexual health and that your nursing care will acknowledge the fact that all of us are unique and special individuals with our own special style of sexual expression.

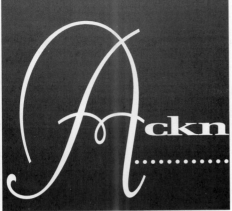

Acknowledgments

Contributors

Lori Cohen-Pasahow, BA, Ob-Gyn Family Planning CNP
Atlantic City Medical Center
Atlantic City, New Jersey

Marian Rudek, RNC, MSN, CRNP
Maternal-Child Health Nurse Practitioner
Shore Memorial Hospital
Somers Point, New Jersey

Al Rundio, PhD, RN, CNAA, CIC
Vice President of Nursing
Adjunct Professor at LaSalle University
Shore Memorial Hospital
Somers Point, New Jersey

Connie Tierno, RN, MS Certified Lactation Consultant
Family Life Specialist
Shore Memorial Hospital
Somers Point, New Jersey

Expert Reviewers

Mary Ellen Florence, PhD, RNCS (Human Sexuality)
Associate Professor of Nursing
Stockton State College
Pomona, New Jersey

Joseph Zawid, MD (Medical Aspects)
Family Practice
Absecon, New Jersey

Part I

An Overview

Chapter 1

Welcome to the World of Human Sexuality

SEX VERSUS SEXUALITY

Ssh…sex. Similarly to other cultures world-wide, the Judaic-Christian culture has difficulty separating the concept of sex from sexuality. This is due to many different doctrines and beliefs. These factors include lack of adequate and accurate sex education from parents and schools, religious, negative childhood sexual experiences, life experiences that may have included childhood sexual trauma and poor relationships with family members, and distorted images and messages from the media.

As a consequence, many men and women do not feel comfortable expressing their sexuality. This is unfortunate, because our sexuality remains with us throughout both health and illness. As nurses we do not typically address sexual concerns because we have not been given the skills and knowledge to talk about them and often feel uncomfortable doing so. For example, how many health professionals do you know who can freely discuss sexual issues? Therefore, one of the main purposes of this book is to increase your comfort level with this topic so that you can be more effective in promoting sexual health.

What is Sexuality?

There are many different facets related to the word *sexuality* because sexuality encompasses all aspects of being and feeling sexual. Unfortunately, many people erroneously think of sexuality only in terms of genital sexual activity, that is, as sex. But sexuality is actually influenced by several different components within a person's life, specifically, by the social, biological, moral, and psychological beliefs and experiences that are part of our development and of our culture's heritage.

The Social Component

Sexuality is influenced by our culture's rules and mores. Mores determine what is societally acceptable within a culture. This may include the meaning and behaviors allowed during dating, what kinds of boy/girl relationships are allowed and who is allowed to marry. Historical influences, which will be discussed in Chapter 2, are also part of this component. Social influences are typically reflected through the media, which frequently define what is considered the "voice" of our culture. Also included within the social component are sex roles. These roles define who we are and how we need to behave to be successful as males and females. Each culture throughout the world has its own unique standards of acceptable sexual behavior.

FIGURE 1—1
The Complexity of Human Sexuality

- Religion
- Ethics
  "Right or Wrong"

- Historical Influences
- Culture-Advertising, TV, Literature
- Relationships
    Family
    Dating
    Marriage

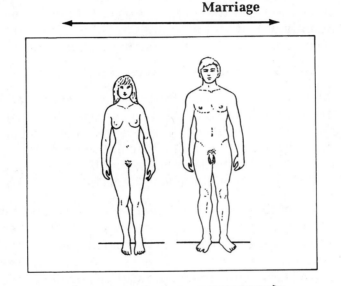

PSYCHOLOGICAL COMPONENT

- Attitudes and Feelings
    About Ourselves
- Family Attitudes
- Past Experiences

BIOLOGICAL COMPONENT

- Growth and Development
- Sexual Response
- Birth Control
    Reproduction
    Pregnancy
    Health

The Psychological Component

Sexuality encompasses learned behavior. We initially "learn" how to act from our family. We decide what is appropriate and valued by observing our parent's behavior. Our parents also send us messages about "clean" and "dirty" and "right" and "wrong". Families frequently teach sexuality via "nonverbal communication." Nonverbal communication can be a powerful communication tool, frequently many of the messages that we have integrated regarding ourselves as sexual beings are related to what our parents don't say in terms of ourselves, our bodies and our actions.

The moral component

Sexuality is interconnected with the psychological component because it is also related to how comfortable we are with others. However, it further encompasses religious beliefs regarding appropriate sexual behavior. What we consider to be "right or wrong" sexually is frequently linked to those religious beliefs. There is a wide diversity of acceptable sexual expression among the many religions of the world.

The biological component

Reproduction, puberty, the physical changes that occur throughout the life cycle, and the physiological changes that occur during the sexual response cycle relate to the biological component of sexuality. This is the component that is usually confused with the broader concept of sexuality. It is also the aspect of sexuality within our culture that we seem to be the most uncomfortable in terms of education and behavior.

Together these four components form the basis of what this book will address for the nurse professional. Since all of these components are interconnected, it would be detrimental to isolate or focus on any one of them alone. It is important that we keep all of these components in mind as we learn to understand how to help patients maintain sexual health.

UNDERSTANDING CONTEMPORARY HUMAN SEXUALITY

It is the author's impression that American cultural attitudes and behaviors regarding sexuality can be characterized by *secrecy*, *ignorance*, and *traumatization*.

Secrecy

Frequently sex is considered a taboo subject; it is "private." This secrecy means that often there is little accurate information that is readily available regarding sexual concerns, behaviors, and experiences. Certain segments of our population such as some teenagers, the illiterate, and those with limited access to reading material and responsible media may not be able to develop an accurate knowledge base to make decisions regarding their sexuality and sexual expression. We are only just becoming aware of the prevalence of sexual abuse and sexual dysfunctions in our culture. In addition, knowledge of contraception is inadequate and often unavailable. This is unfortunate because we are in a period of time when a major new epidemic of sexually transmitted diseases is occurring.

It may be argued that the American media are filled with talk shows that discuss almost every imaginable topic related to sex. These shows, however, typically address the *extremes* of behavior rather than the more common issues experienced by the majority of the population. Despite all the talk, therefore, many Americans have a distorted perception of what is "right" and wrong."

Ignorance

Many patients are also ignorant regarding the social skills necessary to develop good relationships with their mates and their children. As a result of our reluctance to talk about sexuality, this education is missing, and a significant part of the population is basically ignorant regarding such important issues as birth control and the prevention of sexually transmitted diseases.

Statistics suggest that many Americans learn, not through education, but through experience and the consequent pain of this ignorance. For example, in the United States it is believed that more than 1 million teenage girls become pregnant every year. The American teenage birth rate is the highest in the Western Hemisphere; it is double that of Sweden and an astonishing 17 times higher than in Japan. These facts suggest that ignorance is widespread.

Traumatization

Finally, many Americans have been traumatized by the culture. One example of this traumatization is the media's fascination with young, blond, and thin. We are constantly bombarded by such cultural stereotypes. Harold Robbins, Jacqueline Suzanne, and Madonna are all media creations that portray how we should behave and look. Men must be made of steel, and act like machines with unlimited sexual energy, and women must be forever beautiful, blond, and not yet 40.

Since the majority of our patient population do not meet these cultural criteria, such stereotypes generate pain and self-doubt, and these negative emotions will likely affect not only upon how patients feel about themselves sexually, but also their self-esteem in countless other ways. For the disabled and patients with chronic or disfiguring diseases, idealistic stereotypes create even more havoc. Body image changes caused by surgery can cause personal pain and can damage relationships.

Moreover, it is almost impossible to ignore these body changes because the television, which constantly reinforces ideal stereotypes, is usually at the patient's bedside.

Nurses also need to be aware of how these cultural images affect themselves. When we are uncomfortable with an issue or have been traumatized sexually or emotionally during our own lives, we bring our personal history, our cultural diversity, and the consequent feelings of our experiences into our interactions with patients. We therefore need to be aware of the infinite dynamics that contribute to our patients' sense of sexuality and our own sensitivity in addressing these issues.

NURSING AND HUMAN SEXUALITY

Nurses understandably are influenced by the environment in which they live. If this environment is characterized by secrecy, ignorance, and traumatization, it will be difficult for nurses or their patients to discuss sexuality issues. *This is indeed a misfortune, since sexuality is intrinsic to our very being and is one of the most important means of relating to the people and the world around us.*

Despite our culture's stereotypes, societal values are slowly beginning to become more reflective of the diversity and needs of the population, and nurses are in an excellent position to facilitate that change. For example, condoms and information regarding birth control options are now frequently available at school-based health clinics. Nurses *can be* resource agents toward positive change. Nurses can do this by disseminating accurate information regarding sexual health issues, modeling more appropriate ways to communicate about sexuality, and respecting the needs and concerns of their patients by acknowledging all four components of sexuality.

The Role of the Nurse in Human Sexuality

Nursing can trace its roots to almost the beginning of time. However, modern nurses evolved from two distinct groups of people. One of these groups of nurses was composed of medieval monks. English prostitutes, as a means of earning money, also began to care for the sick. Early nursing was therefore carried out by very diverse groups that included both males and females and nurses that were either celibate or highly promiscuous.

In the 19th century, Florence Nightingale prohibited her nurses, who were all women, from wearing jewelry, ornaments, or hair ribbons, and did not allow them to go anywhere unchaperoned. It has been rumored that Ms. Nightingale's students were chosen partly because of their homely looks. This asexual image was maintained for a long time. Although nurses are no longer chosen for school on the basis of their appearance, until recently it was frowned upon for nurses to wear any "unprofessional" ornaments on the uniform, (including pins or earrings). The use of makeup, such as lipstick, was also discouraged.

Before the 1970's, very little information related to human sexuality was published in nursing journals or taught in the classroom. Whether sexuality was to be discussed with the patient was left to the discretion of the physician. In 1973 the World Health Organization studied the curricula of medical and nursing schools and ascertained that little sexual information was being offered in either nursing or medical school. Unfortunately, after a brief attempt to fill this void by adding courses on human sexuality to nursing and medical school curricula, the pendulum has swung back to general silence on these issues.

Compounding this lack of education regarding sexual health are the diverse values present throughout the medical profession. We all bring to our work our own personal values and cultural belief systems. These values influence our professional abilities and our interpretations of what our work should include. Therefore, many nurse professionals cannot comfortably work with every population. One such example of a conflict can be found with the AIDS crisis. Because of religious beliefs, some nurses feel uncomfortable working with the gay population. Another example of value conflict is that of a devout Catholic nurse working in an abortion clinic.

Another major issue for nurses today is the negative sex role discrimination and stereotyping that has characterized the nursing profession. Since 90% of nurses are women, many of the messages related to "how" women should behave and act affect nurses. Society typically views nurses positively as nurturers and caregivers. These two characteristics can be powerful attributes toward positively affecting the healthcare of patients. However, until recently American society frequently also considered nurses to be handmaidens to the male-dominated profession of medicine.

In the 1940s and 50s nurses were portrayed by the media as the paragons of respectability. However, by the 1960s and 1970s the image of nurses had become that of sexual playthings. This is exemplified by get-well cards. These cards frequently show extremely well-endowed young nurses who seem to be exuding sexuality, but possess little intellectual capabilities. Finally, many x-rated movies portray the "promiscuous" woman as a nurse. Thus nurses, unfortunately have become the sexual fantasies of the media. For some nurses this threatening media image may well influence their behavior as they attempt not to be "misread." As a result, they may feel very uncomfortable discussing sexual health concerns with patients. In the 1990s the media frequently characterize nurses in an unrealistic image. Nurses are frequently portrayed as female, single, childless, under thirty-five and only looking for romance and excitement with a physician.

Nurses in our culture cannot help but relate to the mores and belief systems with which they live. However, they need to be aware of how the resulting negative stereotypes may affect how they feel about themselves and how these feeling may affect patient care. And the picture does not have to be so bleak. Nurses have the opportunity to learn and expand their knowledge of human sexuality. As they do so, they can be instrumental in not only questioning but also in changing societal attitudes in a more flexible and accepting manner regarding the diversity of human behavior.

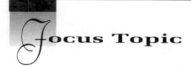

ocus Topic

Definition of Sex and Sexuality

Sex: The word *sex* is most often used in two ways:

1. To label gender, that is, whether a person belongs to the male or female gender or sex.

2. To refer to the physical part of a relationship: intercourse. People use this word in the latter way when they say, "I had sex last night." They are referring to the physical, erotic, or genital relationship.

Sexuality: The word *sexuality* is used to mean something much broader than sex. It refers to the whole person, including his or her thoughts, experiences, learnings, ideas, values, fantasies, and emotions as they have to do with being a male or a female. Sexuality is also related to how we feel about ourselves and how we communicate those feelings to others by the way we act, walk, carry our bodies, talk, and dress. It also includes our interactions and relationships with people of the opposite sex and/or the same sex and how we respond to the messages we receive from them. Sexuality encompasses our lives, from birth to death.

Definitions compiled from the *Family Book About Sexuality* by Mary Calderone, and *Saying Goodbye to the Birds and the Bees: Telling the Real Story* by Nancy Abbey-Harris and Kay Rodenberg Todd.

This definition is the philosophical belief of the author and the premise of this book.

Chapter 2

Sexuality and the Historical Perspective

In order for humanity to survive, men and women procreate. Historically, the interpretations of how, when, and with whom this act should be successfully completed has yielded an enormous amount of confusion, pain, anguish and occasionally pleasure. Consequently, as Chapter 1 has shown, the expression of sexuality is by no means simplistic. Societal messages are complex and can be frequently confusing. Furthermore, within each gender the reality of being male or female has significantly influenced each gender's sexual experience in many different ways.

The cultural attitudes toward sexuality that nurses see derive from our history. Throughout the centuries in every culture there have been diverse and changing attitudes toward what is considered to be appropriate sexual expression.

SOCIAL-HISTORICAL ASPECTS OF SEXUALITY

Because of the diversity of experiences and expectations that characterize the expression of sexuality in different cultures, this overview will be limited to generalizations regarding the Judaic-Christian experience. However, as our world becomes more assimilated and our patients immigrate from all over the world, we need to keep in mind that their expectations and beliefs regarding sexuality may be different than what will be discussed in this chapter. However, the major generalization that emerges from cross cultural studies is that all societies regulate sexual behavior in some way. It is easier to understand present behavior if we understand the roots of that behavior. Patients come to the hospital or other medical care settings with many feelings and experiences regarding sexuality. Unfortunately, many of these feelings are negative and destructive. Bullough, a leading sexologist, wrote that "a major obstacle to understanding our own sexuality is realizing that we are prisoners of past societal attitudes toward sex" (Bullough, 1976, p. xi).

Ancient Roots

Unfortunately, very limited information is available on sexual attitudes, beliefs, and practices before 1000 B.C., and much of that information is derived from art and from the few remaining primitive cultures that still exist today. However, we do know that all cultures have had mores regarding appropriate sex partners. Although the definition of "appropriateness" has changed from culture to culture, incest is a major cultural taboo in every culture.

Prehistoric men and women typically did not understand the link between sex and reproduction. An exception seems to be the ancient Indian religions in the Far East. There is massive evidence that in pre-prehistory the female was extremely valued and worshipped. In fact, female goddesses reigned for 25,000 years before the male gods we all know took over.

The worship of female goddesses may have been due to the fact that during ancient times men and women did not understand the link between intercourse and pregnancy. Therefore, the role of the male in this process was not initially valued. Just how and when human beings learned about the male's role in reproduction is not known, although we estimate that this occurred about 5,000-10,000 years ago.

However it has been speculated that until this knowledge existed, our ancient ancestors may have viewed coitus only as a pleasurable act. With the advent of this knowledge it is likely that men may have achieved more power over women since women no longer could be seen as the only source of life.

Depending upon the culture, various theories of conception were held. Some cultures believed that children were sent by ancestral deities. Other diverse cultural beliefs included: a woman became pregnant by sitting over a fire on which she had roasted a fish received by the prospective father; or that eating human flesh caused pregnancy. In some civilizations it was believed that males could become pregnant.

However, in every culture, both men and women have been aware of their anatomical and physiological differences. It was the woman who menstruated. It was also the woman who became pregnant and who was able to gestate. These observations influenced attitudes and cultural expectations regarding the roles of men and women.

The Beginning of Western Civilization

Among the earliest important cultures in Western civilization were those in Iraq and Egypt (formerly Mesopotamia). Most of the gods worshipped were extensions or representations of nature. These gods symbolized the belief that life was dependent on fertility and thus sex.

In Mesopotamian culture women were viewed with ambivalence. Although they were considered to be low status, owned by men—they could bring life into the world. This ambivalency toward women is reflected in the cults that worshipped the Great Mother.

The Mesopotamians believed that earth was similar to a mother who contained and produced life; a fertile cradle resowing seeds into her womb where they developed into life. However, sometimes this process failed and then people starved. Therefore, the Great Mother was not only worshipped but also feared; and women with their ability to conceive, bear, and nourish life were both feared and revered.

However, the lack of understanding regarding conception and the role of sex in that process endured throughout the era of Greek civilization. The Greek poet Aeschylus believed that a child was conceived by only the sperm of the male. It would be unfair to scoff at these myths because some still exist today. An example of one such myth spoken all too frequently by some of our patients is that "you can't get pregnant by having sex only once."

The ancient Greeks also believed that the first god was a woman named Gaea. Originally Gaea lived alone. However, Gaea became lonely and created for herself a son-cum-lover called Uranus, who represented the sky. Between them they created the rest of all that exists—natural, human, and divine—until Gaea was overthrown by the male Zeus and the Olympians. Another Greek legend is that of the fierce women Amazons, who once a year rode to the borders of their kingdom and had sex with the neighboring tribes. Legend says that they kept any daughters that they had and returned any sons. Almost every ancient culture has myths regarding powerful women. The dominant view however, in Western civilization has been that the female is an insatiably seductive and powerful temptress who can pose danger to the unwitting male. The historical reality is that women's sexuality has usually been under the control of men.

The ancient Greeks were tolerant of, and could even be considered enthusiastic about, male homosexuality. The male body was considered beautiful. Adult men acted as mentors to postpubescent boys and often had homosexual relationships with them. This was a common and approved tradition within the framework of Greek sexual expression. However, there were also restrictive countertrends. Although homosexuality and lesbianism were often tolerated there were periods in both Greek and Roman history where these sexual preferences were severely punished. Moreover, although in the Greek culture there were strong positive feelings regarding marriage and family, women continued to be considered second-class citizens. The Greek stance on women varied from Homeric times to the early Christian period, but in general, the female was clearly subordinate to the male. She was considered to be useful for having children but not as an intellectual companion. However, her sexuality was recognized in a positive way. The great Greek philosopher Aristotle described sexual interactions as natural and believed that both men and women had powerful sexual drives. He felt that orgasm was a pleasurable event for both sexes.

The value of female virginity encouraged early marriage for girls. However, for the male, whose virginity was not an issue, marriage was not encouraged until a much later age. Because wives were typically so much younger than husbands, paternalism, rather than partnership, seemed to be the most influential characteristic of the male/female relationship.

Compared with Greek women, Roman women enjoyed a somewhat higher status. Although they were not equal to their male counterparts, they enjoyed a greater sense of freedom. As Rome became wealthy, this wealth was bestowed by men upon their daughters and wives. To further sexual enhancement, cosmetics and jewelry became an important part of female apparel. Nevertheless, whereas sex was considered one of the pleasures of life for men, for women there were strict standards of acceptable behavior.

The ultimate paradigm of this behavior is the story of Lucretia. Lucretia, a high-ranking Roman woman, killed herself after being raped. This was considered the only honorable ending for a wife who had disgraced her husband. Blame and shame are pervasive behaviors and feelings that are still present for men and women who have been victims of sexual abuse and violence.

The basic source of the Judaic-Christian tradition which is the religious foundation of our Western culture is the Old Testament of the Bible. This is both the source for Judaism and a major component toward the philosophy of Christianity. Basically, there are several important tenets. The Old Testament views sexuality as positive. Sex is a responsibility to God's will. It is a gift.

"So God created man in his own image, in the image of God he created him; male and female he created them." (Genesis 1:27)

Sex was believed to be not just another biological function, but an intimate and important part of a relationship. However, because the Hebrews needed children to continue to exist in the desert, nonprocreative sex was not allowed. Finally, the Old Testament viewed sexual behavior in terms of national and indigenous loyalty.

The ancient Hebrews believed that it was from the male seed alone that an infant developed; women simply provided the warmth, protection, and nutrition of their wombs. Hebrew women were considered to be more or less the same as property, and sexuality and procreation were allowed only in the context of marriage. Among the ancient Hebrews, women were also believed to be more sexual than men. However, their inferior status was clearly reflected in Judaic law. Jewish rules of sexual conduct stressed that adultery was forbidden (Exodus 20:13). Among the Hebrews only *married* women could be guilty of adultery; that is, adultery referred only to a married woman's having sexual intercourse with a man other than her husband. When a man had sex with a woman who was married to someone else he was only charged with the violation of the husband's property rights. Although he too was punished, unlike the woman, he was not punished by death.

However, since the ancient Jews also believed that there was an inherent pleasure in sex, sex was also considered a right of married women. Consequently, any male who could not, by reasons of impotence or his profession, satisfy his wives' needs could be divorced. Judaism itself was a male-oriented religion with considerable ambiguity toward women. This ambiguity is reflected in Jewish Talmudic scripture, consistent with the belief system of prior cultures, where women are considered to have a more constant and aggressive sexual drive than men. For example, it was Eve who led Adam astray (Genesis 3:1-6) Despite the fear of their aggressiveness, women were subordinate to men.

In general, then, the early civilizations of the world suggest a strong and powerful position for men but not for women. Though cultures differed, women seem in general to have lived and experienced sexuality through the context and comfort of male interpretation and approval. These attitudes toward male and female sexuality will become even more evident as we discuss Christianity and its influence on American culture.

Christianity and the Middle Ages

The world in which Christianity developed was one of tremendous controversy in terms of philosophy, religion and morality. Christian attitudes derived from a combination of Greek, Jewish, and current beliefs of that time such as dualism. Many cults existed, often characterized by some form of *dualism*. Dualism is the belief that the body and spirit were unalterably separate and opposed to each other. The goal of Christian life was to become purely spiritual. This was done by transcending both the material and physical aspects of life.

In the Christian theological view, women were seen as the repository of lust, the door to the devil. Furthermore, women were the initiators of guilt and the enticers of men. This attitude was epitomized by St. Paul who, like the Hebrews, believed that Eve was the catalyst to Adam's fall. His beliefs led to the Doctrine of the Strict Subjugation of Women, which reinforced women's inferiority. In fact, it was believed that when women were in the presence of men the only appropriate behavior for them was to act hesitant. As late as the ninth century, serious debate arose over whether women had souls. In fact, the early medieval clergy blamed behaviors such as impatience and loss of memory on women. These physical conditions were viewed as being caused by the devil and his allies, female wenches.

In the early Christian view, women could only be saved through the process of childbirth and through the continuity of faith, charity, and holiness toward God (1 Timothy 1:11-15).

The Christian religious leaders were not unaware of the difficulty of sexual abstinence. St. Paul stated that although "it is good for a man not to touch a woman...it is better to marry than to burn" (1 Corinthians 7:1-12). This belief system helped encourage the attitude of sex only within marriage.

By the end of the fourth century the church held a rigid negative view regarding sexual expression. Although St. Augustine as a youth led a life full of sexual experiences, he changed his philosophy when he grew older, and his views exerted a tremendous influence upon the Christian attitude that sexual lust was evil and that this inherent lust separated humanity from closeness with God. Pope Leo IX (1048-1054) formally ended clerical marriage and commanded celibacy for all priests. Except for sex for procreation, sex was strongly condemned. This attitude of repression is still found in contemporary times.

Over the next 16 centuries sexual attitudes, morals, and behavior patterns were like a pendulum, swinging back and forth between permissiveness and repression. Around the 12th century courtly love evolved from the Christian experience of repression. This was a new concept, practiced by the upper class, which defined acceptable or appropriate sexual behavior in terms of romanticism, secrecy, and valor. "Pure" love was viewed as different from; and incongruent with, physical love. One expression or "trial" of this "love" was through the ritual of lovers testing their allegiance to one another by lying in bed together without having sex. This act was believed to prove the purity of their love.

In the 15th century chastity belts appeared. They served two purposes. These belts were developed to protect women from rape when their husbands were away at war. But women, much like money and other valuables, were also perceived to be the "property" of their husbands who were worried that during their long absences their wives and daughters would not only be sought after but would actively seek the pleasures of other men. Chastity belts were a way to protect their property.

After courtly love faded, sexual behavior became less romantic and more physical in expression. A sense of increased permissiveness appeared with the emergence of the Protestant Reformation in the 16th century and reversed many of the repressive Roman Catholic doctrines. Indeed, the clergy could marry. Lay people were even allowed to enjoy sex as long as they adhered to the Protestant work ethic.

However, the Protestants were also somewhat ambivalent. Martin Luther, who was the leading force behind the Reformation is a good example of the conflict. Although he warned of the consequences of masturbation and lustful thoughts, he renounced his own vows of celibacy to marry.

During the Renaissance, in the 16th and 17th century, "romantic love" again flourished throughout Europe as the Dark Ages came to an end. Literature, painting, and the theater emphasized "wine, women, and song." However, the pendulum soon swung back to severe repression as the devastating epidemic of syphilis swept out of Genoa, Italy, to cover the entire European continent with the "large pox."

Sexual behavior in the 18th and 19th century was characterized by broad ranges of what was deemed appropriate. In general, however, European culture was much less repressive than American Puritan culture, which held strong ideals for family life and therefore condemned adultery and premarital sex.

Early American Attitudes

When the early European colonists arrived in North America, as many as 1 million American Indians lived there. Although Indian customs varied greatly, in general, unmarried Indian women were afforded a great amount of sexual freedom, whereas married women were expected to remain faithful to their husbands. As more European men came to America, marriage with Indian women occurred with greater frequency. In 1556 several laws were passed in English and Spanish colonies legitimizing such marriages. The Indian population was soon joined by both bonded and free European men and women, as well as by African men and women brought here as slaves. However, as the population grew to be more dominantly European, it was the European values that tried to control and dictate sexuality and morality.

Early Puritan Calvinists fleeing from England brought with them their beliefs that men and women were sinful by nature. They viewed marital sex as a necessary evil and nonmarital sex as something to be avoided. Clergymen, like early Christian spokesmen, frequently portrayed women as the dangerous embodiments of Eve, or as temptresses. Throughout the 17th century there was also a common belief in the existence of witches. A witch was frequently accused of having sexual relations with the devil. However, when Cotton and Increase Mather were put on trial for improperly "laying on of hands" in exorcising a naked 17-year-old girl, hundreds of other women suspected of being witches were released. This seemed to end the witch hunts of early America.

However, historians have found a discrepancy between the Puritans' stated values and their actual behavior. For instance, premarital sex, adultery, illegitimacy, rape, and, to a lesser extent, homosexuality were widespread. This behavior may have been the result of the disproportionate male/female ratio, which was close to 30 males for every female. The scarcity of women also encouraged prostitution, which was perceived by the Church to be a major problem in early America. Another common behavior was bestiality. Sexual abuse of sheep, goats, and calves were common among male colonists.

Sexuality in the middle colonies was more relaxed. In New York and Pennsylvania, among groups like the Pennsylvania Dutch, premarital sex was an accepted social custom. Because of the rights of ownership, white men were able to have considerable sexual liberties with black slave women and white indentured slaves. It was not uncommon for white men to have long-lasting relationships with their black slaves. In the southern colonies sexuality was influenced by slavery and the less rigid Anglican church. A sexual double standard also existed between men and women. Many white men openly kept black slaves and white servant women as mistresses. The southern white woman was not allowed those kinds of relationships or pleasures with black men. In fact, accusations of such contact frequently resulted in the imprisonment or death of the black male slave. The word "paradox" seems well suited to a description of the 18th century. That is because although religion was fervently practiced and condoned, premarital sex, illegitimacy and nonconsenting sex with slaves and servants was allowed and even condoned.

The 18th and 19th Centuries

American culture became more diversified in its sexual attitudes as it began to reach out into the frontier. In the West, with women scarce, men lonely, and almost no control from the Church or governing bodies, prostitution became very common. Homosexuality and bestiality were also common in the West.

European culture had a somewhat dissimilar experience due to Queen Victoria. Victoria reigned in England from 1837-1901. She imagined herself not only to be a military leader, but also a moral leader. In response to what she felt was excessive sexual behavior in England, she slowly began to modify the behavior of its citizens. *Victorianism* named after the Queen, is a term used to depict an inhibited attitude toward sexuality that stresses modesty and innocence. Victorianism succeeded in convincing generations of men and women that sexuality was dirty. These attitudes quickly spread to America. It became "indelicate" to offer a lady a leg of chicken, clothing literally covered women from head to toe, piano legs were covered with crinolines, and even books by authors of the opposite sex were frequently placed on different bookshelves.

However, many double standards appeared along with the ideal of modesty. For example, the wealthy frequently had secret mistresses. Another flip side of the repressive behavior was pornography, which became rampant, and prostitution, which became legalized in Europe. Victorian morality was indeed a privilege of the "upper" class. Indeed a double standard existed between the behaviors o the upper and lower classes. For example, upper class women were not supposed to enjoy sex, whereas female prostitution among the lower classes flourished due to the patronage of upper class men. Once again, sexual behavior for the upper class was judged by different standards than that of the masses.

Americans also attempted to copy what was seen as sexually correct in Victorian England. Legs became "limbs," breasts were called "bosoms," being pregnant was "anceinte," and masturbation was called "the solitary vice." At the same time, science and the field of medicine became important leaders in judging what was "healthy" or "abnormal" sexuality. Many misleading myths were formed. For example, masturbation was thought to cause brain damage, and women were viewed as having little capacity for sexual enjoyment. Perhaps the most enduring legacy of the Victorian era may be the strongly held belief that in all matters that are considered to be sexual, ignorance is best.

The early 20th century also saw the beginning of the "medicalization" of sexuality. Publications appeared on "sexual physiology" and "sexual hygiene," as well as on obstetrical care. Books written by men, for women, on the medical and sexual experiences of women presented women as "congenitally incapable of experiencing complete sexual satisfaction" (Ellis, 1903) and as not being capable of having natural childbirth without male medical obstetrical interventions. Another typical attitude was voiced by a very popular sex expert, William Acton (1865): "As a general rule, a modest women seldom desires sexuality or sexual gratification for herself. She submits to her husband, but only to please him; and, but for the desire of maternity, would far rather be relieved from his attention." This mentality, which perceives women as either madonnas or whores, is still one part of today's mythology.

Another instrumental force toward perpetuating sexual discomfort and modesty was concern about controlling, timing, and limiting pregnancy. Thomas Malthus inspired the beginning of the birth control movement by advocating sexual restraint and late marriage. Since coitus interruptus was considered "dangerous" to mental health, and the rhythm method was considered equally unreliable, many of the popular advice books urged couples to restrain from sex. Pregnancy was also increasingly "medicalized" as well as the disappearance for the upper class of midwives.

These practices had effects on female sexuality. For example, it was believed that simultaneous orgasm increased the possibility of conception. Since large families with as many as 15 or 20 children were not uncommon and childbirth was a perilous, often life-threatening experience, orgasm was not always seen as worth the perils of multiple pregnancies.

Finally, venereal disease was a major problem throughout America. It is estimated that as much as 30% of the population had either syphilis or gonorrhea. In an era before the time of penicillin, sexually transmitted diseases were justifiably feared by the population.

The Late 19th and Early 20th Centuries

From the later part of the 19th century through the 20th century, some of these ideas changed as other philosophical feelings about sexuality and women's control of their bodies began to develop and influence sexuality. The founder of modern sexology is Kraft-Ebbing. His book Psychopathia Sexualis (1886), which undertook a detailed classification of sexual disorders, set the attitude for how specific sexual behaviors would be viewed in the coming century. Although he advocated sympathetic medical tolerance for patients with sexual deviations, his descriptions of their behaviors were so graphic that he scared many people and inadvertently created intolerance in the population at large.

Sigmund Freud (1856-1939) also influenced how we would view and react to ourselves as sexual beings. Although he is recognized as the father of psychotherapy, his most important medical contribution may have been his identification of the importance of sexuality in human existence. Freud emphasized the centrality of sex in every aspect of human development.

Freud believed that all behaviors were a reaction to, and motivation for, sexual expression. He also believed that sexuality was the cause of what we term "neurosis." He identified and wrote about sexuality in infants and children, and developed a theory of psychosexual development which will be discussed in a later chapter on children and sexuality.

Freud also described the Oedipal and Electra complexes, which describe the love that the child holds for the parent of the opposite sex. According to Freud, for little boys, this love may be "dangerous." To avoid their father's anger, little boys must give up their first love object, their mother, and identify with their father. Little girls also experience love for both parents, and they too must give up their love for one parent. Little girls must give up their love for their father and continue to identify with their mother. Freud believed that this task affects men and women throughout their lives.

Freud developed certain important concepts regarding the essential components of sexuality. *Castration anxiety* means fear of having the penis cut off because of inappropriate sexual feelings for the mother. *Penis envy*, another concept developed by Freud, describes how little girls grow up feeling envious and inferior because they do not have a penis. Although some of what Freud postulated is disputed in contemporary times, his work and philosophy had a profound impact upon Western culture.

The actual study of human sexuality began flourishing in the late 19th and early 20th century with the appearance of a group now termed *sexual scientists*. Havelock Ellis, an English psychologist, author, and physician, published a seven-volume collection, Studies *in the Psychology of Sex* (1903). Within this massive work Ellis discussed the fact that women were not only as interested in sex as men but were even more sexual than men. The reason is that female arousal includes several body parts, such as the clitoris, the breast, the vagina, and the uterus, whereas male sexuality primarily focuses on the penis. Ellis further stated that women might be more psychologically interested in sex than men because of their greater physiological response. Unfortunately for women, he also wrote, "In a certain sense their brains are in their wombs" (1903). Needless to say, feminists were quite incensed with his remarks.

Between 1900 and 1953 public discussion and scholarly writing advocating more liberal attitudes regarding sexuality increased. This change in philosophy was exemplified in manuals that advocated pleasure rather than simply procreation. However, pleasure was condoned only within the context of marriage. A unique example of one such early 20th-century manual was written by Dr. Helena Wright, a female gynecologist. Dr. Wright included a step-by-step instruction guide to help women achieve orgasm through intercourse, as well as a guide to masturbation. She believed that female sexual desire had slowly become "acceptable" because it was considered dependent upon on the husband to activate it. Finally, she believed that female sexuality was also more spiritual and pure than the purely physical sexuality of men. In a sense Dr. Wright can be considered to be an encourager of the expression of female sexuality.

Contemporary American Culture

One of the first scientists who attempted to study sexuality was Alfred Kinsey. The Kinsey report (1953) had a major impact upon our understanding of sexuality in the United States. Kinsey interviewed a total of 5,300 males and 5,940 females and published the results in his volumes: *Sexual Behavior in the Human Male* and *Sexual Behavior in the Human Female*. Kinsey can be credited with empowering Americans to talk more openly about sex. He was the "permission" giver who empowered people to begin to talk about sexual behavior. One of his contributions was the Kinsey Scale, which rated sexual orientation on a 1 to 7 score. Kinsey also found that 50% of married men and 26% of married women had had previous affairs, or, as people came to say, "at least one bridge player in a table of four." Another finding was that sexual functioning seemed to peak at the age of 30 for women and at 16 or 17 for men.

Another monumental achievement was the publication of *Human Sexual Response* (1964) by Masters and Johnson. For the first time a precise understanding of the biology of the sexual response cycle was achieved. From this base the authors developed sex therapy for the common sexual problems such as impotence and premature ejaculation. In 1977, Helen Singer Kaplan added another dimension to the response cycle by identifying "desire" as a necessary component of sexual functioning.

The 20th century and the sexual behavior of this generation have also been influenced by several other sociological and scientific factors, some of which occurred earlier. These included (1) the Industrial Revolution, (2) advances in medicine which changed the life expectancy from 47 to almost 80 years of age, (3) the development of the birth control pill, which allowed men and women to enjoy sexuality without the fear of pregnancy, (4) the sexual revolution, which was a partial response to the development of the pill, and finally (5) radio, TV, motion pictures, and VCRs, which brought every aspect of sexuality into the home.

The revolution of contraception occurred as a result of the birth control pill. For the first time procreation could effectively be separated from recreational sex. This had significant implications not only for individuals but also for religious institutions and social arenas, and we are not always comfortable with many of the issues that the pill has forced us to confront. For example, although teenagers now have access to birth control, not all teenagers (or adults) have the necessary decision-making skills to address the responsibilities that are needed when being sexually active. Parents also fear that the "pill" increases promiscuity.

The birth control pill has also brought with it an increase in sexually transmitted diseases. As nurses you may well have to do counseling and nursing care regarding how to prevent and also treat these diseases. With the advent of AIDS, sexually transmitted diseases have once again significantly increased mortality. A further consequence is increased infertility as a result of scarred fallopian tubes. This can be caused by several different sexually transmitted diseases.

The timing of our rites of passage has also changed as a result of better health care. One such change that health care professionals may be forced to confront is earlier puberty. For instance, in 1850 puberty occurred at the age of 16; now it occurs for most children at the age of 12. Similarly, the original time span of adolescence which was once 2 to 4 years, has now been extended to more than 10 years. Delaying sexuality for 10 years until marriage is no longer realistic for many young people. Another example of change is the age of the first marriage. In

1850 marriage typically occurred at the age of 18. Today, marriages do not usually occur until people reach the age of 22 to 23.

Extended life expectancy creates another challenge to our coping skills regarding sexuality. In 1900 the average age of death was 47, and the average marriage typically lasted 20 to 25 years. Usually one marital partner died approximately 4 years after the last child left home. Today the average life expectancy is closer to 80, and hypothetically a marriage could last 50 years. How can couples keep their marriages sexually exciting or satisfying for so many years? As health professionals and more generally as participants in a wider culture, we have developed few skills to help people live happily in a long marriage. In some cases spouses may be forced to care for and make decisions for mates that they are no longer close to or with whom they have lacked intimacy for many years.

The decades of the 1960s and 70s introduced to American culture many changes and conflicts, including a sexual revolution. This revolution dramatically changed the mores and behavior of a large majority of our population as it challenged the notion of many of our long-established sexual beliefs. Sex for recreational purposes, gender role issues, challenges to the notion of the traditional marriage, abortion rights, and the concept of "make love not war" were introduced.

These changes affected the way that men and women acted out their sexuality. Sex was no longer viewed as something to be enjoyed only within the context of marriage. Sex roles, or the roles that men and women play not only in marriage but in every aspect of their lives, were challenged. For many, androgyny, or the existence of both male and female behavioral characteristics within a person, became a goal.

With these changes, women have become more challenged, and many women have fallen into the trap of becoming superwomen to themselves and their families. As a result, many of the women patients that you may see have tremendous responsibilities that include family and professional concerns. Men also have conflicts regarding their sex roles because they are now being challenged to become more caring and sensitive.

These changes have triggered conflicts for both men and women as they strive to develop reasonable expectations regarding male and female roles. For example, positive sexual expression is a very new experience in women's history. As a result, not all women have acquired the skills or the ability to competently address sexual issues.

Nurses can be excellent role models for their patients but to do this they must be aware of their own cultural influences, biases, and beliefs regarding male and female sexuality. Although the pendulum has swung back somewhat since the changes of the 1960's, but is more liberal than the 1980s, we as a culture in the 1990s have become slightly more conservative. Many of the original conflicts that this revolution introduced are still being experienced by not only your patients but probably by yourselves. Issues such as abortion, access to sex education, sexual harassment, equality for women, and child protection laws are all problematic.

Everyone in our culture is living in an era of tremendous sociological change. These changes can cause ambivalent and conflicting attitudes which may well affect the practice of nursing and what patients expect and ask of you. As noted earlier, the notion of what is "right or wrong" sexually changes almost constantly and may be a constant source of stress and ambivalence for your patient. As nurses it is very important that we are aware of the emotional turmoil that these issues evoke in ourselves and in our patients.

Hopefully the 1990s will be an era that is characterized by a deeper and more powerful expression of, and enjoyment of sexuality.

Part II

Sexuality and the Life Cycle

A baby lies in her mother's arms. She smiles contentedly. The mother begins to stroke the baby's body. She rubs the baby's neck and arms, and holds her close to her breast. Mother smiles contentedly as the baby nestles in her arms. The baby's body feels good. The stimulation that her mother creates in her skin is one way of being attached and connected to mother. It is also the way that she begins to perceive and decode messages regarding her body, pleasure, and the nature of relationships. It is the beginning of putting her in touch with sexuality. She is a sexual being.

The couple have been waiting for the baby to go to sleep. Finally, they no longer hear the stirrings of their child as she settles into a sleep that will keep her comfortable until her hunger wakens her. The parents snuggle together and begin to make love. Their lovemaking consists of both erotic sexual movements and sexual intercourse. They smile at one another. At this moment they are lovers. They become very intense in giving each other pleasure. After a while they feel satisfied. Mother, father, and baby are all asleep. The house is quiet.

She is 40 and the mother of three children. For the past 8 years she has also been a single mother. Her husband left when he felt overwhelmed with the responsibilities of a family. Of course, his alcoholism didn't help him cope with their needs. Today, after work, she went to a Little League game, did her food shopping and made dinner. Finally, all is quiet in the house. Slowly she goes to her room, takes a bath, and carefully applies her moisturizing cream. She puts on the television. The actor is very good looking. She closes her eyes and begins to fantasize herself in his arms. She is a sexual being.

An elderly man of 80 lies in his lover's arms. His body is frail and his health is no longer good. He is plagued with chronic disease. The couple smile contentedly as they massage and hug one another. They share a private joke and there is laughter. Although, because of diabetes, he can no longer have an erection, they look forward to this quiet and loving time together. They are sexual beings.

Although these are unique scenarios, these people are all sexual beings. The expression of sexuality is a human desire that is intrinsic throughout the entire life cycle. Even as its "mechanism" and expression change as the life cycle advances or relationships change, sexuality remains an inherent part of the health of our patients and of ourselves. As already noted, it is believed that we are sexual beings from almost the time of conception, and we still have the potential for sexual expression as we come to the end of our lives.

Nurses can help patients by being aware of the major developmental, psychosocial and medical issues that both negatively and positively can affect the expression of sexuality throughout the life cycle. The following chapters therefore review the important changes that typically occur throughout the transition points of the life cycle.

Welcome to the World: Childhood Sexuality

For some people, the thought of children as sexual beings may cause high levels of anxiety and even denial. For adults who may have been victims of childhood sexual abuse, this topic may be impossible to process in any way other than with terror or fear. However, for the majority of adults, childhood experiences of sexuality have been non-traumatic and even positive.

Although childhood sexuality is an important concept to understand and acknowledge, the sexual expression of children is rarely a concern on the medical floor of a hospital. Nevertheless, well or sick, a child is a sexual being. The attitudes of those who care for children can have a long-term impact upon children's self-esteem and their ease in expressing sexuality.

This chapter discusses the physical changes and interpsychic demands and adaptations necessary to become healthy, mature sexual beings. It includes an overview of the major developmental theories on small children put forth by Sigmund Freud, Erik Erikson, and Margaret Mahler. (See Focus Topic starting on page 56.) It also identifies some of the medical challenges that may confront your young patient's sexuality.

PRENATAL PERIOD

The uterus is the holding environment in which dramatic physical changes occur for the fetus. Within this environment of warmth and security the infant's sexual development proceeds both externally and internally. The presence or omission of the Y chromosome differentiates the female from the male. Females have an XX chromosome pattern, and males have an XY chromosome pattern.

Even in utero little boys have erections. Although these are purely physiological (autoerotic), this response can be viewed as preparation for the time when the little boy leaves the safety of his mother's body and ventures into the world. In fact, nocturnal penile tumescence can occur as frequently as three times a day as the male fetus prepares to enter the world. It has also been hypothesized that little girls may have vaginal lubrication *in utero*, though obviously this is very hard to observe.

INFANCY

Developmental Challenges

Once infants enter the world, a new set of experiences and demands awaits them.

In the first 6 months of life newborn infants cannot differentiate between themselves and their mother. According to *object-relations theory*, this is known as the *autistic phase of development.* Object-relations theory evolved from the psychoanalytic work of Freud, Winnicott, Fairbairn and several other theorists.

Margaret Mahler explored the development of the child in relationship to its mother through the stages of separation and individuation. Psychologists hidden behind a glass window observed the interactions of mothers and their small infants in a nursery setting in England. The resulting theory, a kind of extension of Freudian theory, is based on the hypothesis that we create mental images of significant others, such as mother. This is accomplished via the "ego" which is capable of relating to an external object.We then use these images to define for ourselves a sense of good and bad people. These initial relationships are the basis for the development of a healthy, well-functioning ego. This theory holds that the human infant is capable of reacting fully from birth.

However, during this early phase of development children have no sense of the boundaries of their body. Those who are deprived of maternal stimulation during this stage, such as holding, hugging, and eye contact, may grow up to be profoundly disturbed and even autistic.

Mentally, newborn infants also have no way of differentiating experiences. It is basically with an all-or-nothing response that they perceive the world. Whatever stimuli are felt most strongly, will be the ultimate perceived events. Infants are therefore at the mercy of those who care for them and have no resources to rationalize or understand any experience. At this stage of life, according to Freud's anatomy of the personality, the baby is all *id,* or primitive impulses.

The early months of life exert an enormous influence upon childrens' perception of the world. Will it feel safe or will it feel unsafe and unpredictable? These perceptions are influenced by the mother or the primary caregiver. One of the first ways that an infant begins to relate to the world is through the "eyes" of the mother. Making eye contact with the mother also begins to precipitate the social smile.

Similarly, feelings about sexuality begin to form in these early months. Freud used the word **sexual** to include not only genital sexuality but also the pregenital drive. According to Freud's theory of psychosexual development, this period of sexual development is known as the *oral stage*. The mouth serves a dual purpose: it not only helps satiate the infant but is also a means of expressing aggressive impulses.

During the oral stage infants express all of their needs through their mouth. Survival is based on the development of the sucking reflex. Infants also sense the love and security of their mother through their mouth. The skin is another organ that helps them sense the world. First the mouth, then the eyes, and finally the hands bring the child into muscular competence.

Erik Erikson, a leading human developmentalist, developed a psychosocial model of human development based on tasks that needed to be accomplished throughout the life cycle. Erikson believed that during each phase of life certain intrapsychic issues had to be successfully resolved. If the tasks related to these issues were not accomplished successfully, the individual would be affected emotionally in a very negative way. These stages have been popularly called the "eight stages of man."

The first stage facing the infant is to resolve the issue of *trust versus mistrust*. This is achieved through the infant's first relationship. If this relationship is successful, the world and the people in it can be viewed as safe and happy. Without trust the individual will be unable to form healthy relationships.

The mother is typically the basis for the development of trust: She is the first source of pleasure and love, as well as the first source of anguish, frustration, and fear. Although fathers are also important, it is the mother who is usually of primary importance.

Experience of Sexuality

Infant males experience sexual sensations from the time of birth because their genitalia are exposed and susceptible to stimulation. Infants can frequently be quieted by genital stroking and tickling. This is a common behavior in many cultures. In the United States most parents are uncomfortable with it, as are probably many health professionals.

Other sources of genital stimulation are available for the infant every day. Diaper changing, cleansing of the genitals, and even rubbing of lotions on the body to care for diaper rash can elicit pleasure. Although they are less likely to have inadvertent stimulation, baby girls also experience genital sensations through daily caregiving . There has been speculation about whether baby girls are aware of their vagina, and recent research seems to suggest that little girls indeed feel genital stimulation. Observations also show that almost as soon as physical coordination develops, little girls will insert their fingers into their vaginas.

It has also been observed that as early as 4 weeks of age infants can experience orgasm. Once they are able to identify which body parts feel good to touch, infants will frequently masturbate. Although for many parents this is a cause for great concern, it cannot be overemphasized that this is normal behavior.

Vision is also an important sexual development tool because it is one of the principal means by which infants organize their world. The visibility of the male sexual organs and the lack of this visibility in little girls seem to influence the sense of difference between boys and girls. This awareness is one of the initial ways in which infants can identify themselves. Male infants also seem to be very aware of the changes that occur in their penis. In little girls these sensations seem to be less genitally focused.

Although there has been controversy regarding sex differences between baby boys and girls, some differences may be noticed. Little boys tend to be more muscular and are sometimes more irritable. Baby girls seem to cry less and sleep more. However, these are broad generalizations and may be linked to socialization. Those of us who have had cranky girls and calm boys will be sure to disagree with these generalizations.

Implications for Nursing

One of the most significant tasks beginning during the second 6 months of life and extending through infancy is learning to differentiate self from other. As children mature, they begin to differentiate·themselves from their caregivers. This process may take as long as 2 years. As reviewed, according to object-relations theory, this is known as the *separation-individuation period* of life. During this time infants become increasingly aware of their surroundings and their caregivers. Initially they can only identify mother. However, as they begin to differentiate mother, strangers become alarming, unsafe beings. Therefore, infants in a hospital setting or in any setting in which they will be separated from mother or need to come into contact with strangers typically feel very threatened and anxious. Keeping the child as close as possible to mother is crucial to the child's sense of security and well-being.

EARLY CHILDHOOD

Developmental Challenges

Early childhood occurs between the ages of approximately 2 to 5 years. During this period, enormous developmental demands are placed upon the child.

Freud termed the first part of this period the *anal stage*. He theorized that this stage of pregenital sexuality was characterized by conflict between two modes of behavior: retention and elimination, or between learning to "let go" and "holding on." During the anal stage children also need to learn to increase their independence and to gain mastery over their body functions. They need to learn to say yes or no, to love, to give, to withhold, and even to hate.

A major developmental conflict for the child is toilet training. This can be either a positive or negative experience for both child and parent. If the parents are too rigid in enforcing this training, they may well find themselves in a battle with their toddler. Toddlers may experience a great sense of mastery if this experience is positive and has been done in a gentle, caring way. Other Children may have a sense of loss because they must learn to conform to the world around them and no longer have the unconditional love of the parent.

The hospital setting can be very confusing for children who are going through toilet training or have just been trained. They may feel very shamed if they are now given a diaper or if they need to be catheterized. Basically, any touching or "invasion" into their body can be traumatic. They may also feel confusion that strangers are now touching their genitals.

For many children, the hospital experience is a time of immense regression. They will revert back to more infantile behavior. Therefore, whenever possible, it is important to allow children to hold on to whatever mastery they have accomplished. It is also very important to allow them to participate in their care.

Nurses should also explain to children what is going to occur, and be as honest as possible. The child may feel unsafe. We need to give the child whatever coping tools we can to help with the experience of hospitalization or of even just getting health care.

Freud also believed that during this period of time the *ego* is more fully beginning to develop. The *ego* is the conscious part of the brain that helps moderate behavior, including the primitive impulses of the *id*. One of the first tasks of the emerging ego is to help children learn to conform. Another task is to help them differentiate between appropriate and inappropriate behavior.

Erik Erikson called the conflict of this second developmental stage the conflict between *autonomy versus shame*. He believed that the small child needs a sense of graded independence. For example, toddlers begin to learn to develop a sense of self-reliance and adequacy as their communication skills increase. As they reach out and their mobility increases, they gain a sense of power and mastery. This mastery is frequently tested by the temper tantrums so commonly encountered during this age. Without these successes a sense of shame may develop.

According to Erikson, another third developmental stage of this early childhood period is that of *initiative versus guilt*. As children learn more about the world and the people in it, they must learn how to assert themselves without feeling inferior or guilty. During this stage they are great imitators of their parents, and they also learn how to start to make decisions for themselves. If successful during this stage, children should become more self-assured and confident regarding the world around them.

Sexuality

At around 3 years of age little boys and girls become more concretely aware of the genitals and the pleasure that they can have by manipulating them. The "zones" that are associated with libido are the penis and the clitoris.

The *Oedipus complex* and the *Electra complex* are terms derived from the psychosexual theories of Freud. Freud believed that little boys fall in love with their mothers and develop a deep rivalry with their fathers for the love of the mother. However, because their fathers are more powerful, little boys become fearful that their father will castrate them for falling in love with mother. Further reinforcing this concern is the recognition that little girls and their mothers do not have a penis. To repress these fears, small boys begin to identify with their fathers and repress their sexual interest in their mothers.

Freud believed that little girls also fall in love with their fathers. He postulated that for the female child the clitoris was the equivalent of a small penis, and that in the oral and anal stages sexuality was masculine, or phallic, for both boys and girls. Little girls "discover" that boys have a penis because it is more visible. According to Freud, the penis is perceived as superior to the clitoris. The little girl then develops "penis envy" and a feeling of having been castrated. This "penis envy" results in the little girl wanting to possess her father and to replace her mother, whom she blames for her dilemma. However, this is a "hopeless love" and the little girl must learn to repress this love. One mechanism that she will use to resolve this dilemma is to begin to identify with mother. Freud termed this developmental experience the Electra complex (the Electra complex was named after a Greek legend about a princess that helped kill her mother).

Although Freud's theories have been disputed by many, some of the basic premises may be accurate: the first love objects of little boys are most likely their mothers and the first love objects of little girls are usually their fathers. Eventually, if development continues without any problems, small children bury these conflicts in their unconscious.

According to Freud's theory of psychosexual development, at approximately 4 years of age children enter the *phallic stage*, or the stage of early pregenital sexuality. The phallic stage is characterized by the crucial task of consolidating his or her sexually differentiated body image, renouncing the sex role not appropriate to his or her own sex, and accepting the indefinite postponement of full genital functioning. This is also the time when many of the child's self-concepts become solidified. Attitudes formed during this period are crucial for later heterosexual development.

Some believe that Erikson's and Freud's theories are limited because they were both based on a male developmental model. Furthermore, Freud was a citizen of his time: the Victorian era, during which males were viewed as more powerful and more psychologically healthy than females. The works of Carol Gilligan, Nancy Chodorow, and other contemporary feminist psychologists are strongly challenging these earlier psychosocial and psychosexual presumptions regarding male and female development. There is a growing consensus among feminist scholars that the female self, more so than the male, is defined by its relation to others, especially its family of origin. Therefore little girls should not be viewed as emotionally "immature or weaker" but rather be acknowledged that they possess different qualities than little boys.

Sexual Identity

Another very important concept to comprehend in understanding childhood sexuality is sexual identity. There are three areas of behavior that incorporate sexual identity: core gender identity, sex roles, and sexual orientation.

Core Gender Identity

This includes the concept of "I am a boy" or "I am a girl." This awareness is typically established by the time that native language develops, but it may occur as early as the delivery room, when it is loudly announced, "It's a boy" or "It's a girl!" Core gender identity seems to be firmly internalized by the age of 18 months. Once this sense of identity is established, it is almost impossible to change.

Children who do not develop a typical gender identity will feel that they are trapped in the wrong gender body. As adults they may be called *transsexuals*. Although there are many different theories as to why someone develops a *gender dysphoria*, we are not very clear about the etiology of this disorder.

Sex Roles

These include all of the behaviors that are associated with being boys or girls. Although sex role behavior today is not as rigidly defined as in previous generations, our culture still attaches many expectations to gender. Research has shown that there is a strong societal bias that perpetuates the belief that boys and girls are emotionally different.

For example, little boys and girls are frequently given toys that reinforce appropriate sex role behavior. This behavior becomes very apparent after the age of 3 and is greatly influenced by parental behavior and attitude. Research has shown that girls are typically held and cuddled more than boys and boys are more frequently roughhoused.

Whatever their cause, basic personality differences do seem to occur. Some of these differences are expressed by the degree of comfort with certain behaviors. Women's comfort with, or perhaps acceptance of, the responsibility of child care may contribute to their predisposition to defining themselves in terms of relationships. Empathy, which is defined as a feminine characteristic, seems to be easily expressed by little girls.

For boys and men, separation and individuation seem to be tied to gender identity, since separation from their mother is necessary for the development of male sex role behavior. Since feminine sex role behavior does not depend upon this separation, it has been theorized that because little girls do not have to experience this traumatic separation, they can be more comfortable expressing all of those characteristics that are viewed as "girl" behavior, such as nurturing and being loving, expressive, and dependent. It has been further theorized that boys, however, must "learn to be boys" if they are to successfully negotiate separating from mother and becoming similar to father: that is, to be strong, rough, and never to cry or be too expressive.

Gradually stereotypes regarding expected sex role behavior are changing. Boys are slowly being allowed to be expressive, and girls are slowly being encouraged to be independent and assertive. Stereotypes regarding what is "boy" or "girl" behavior is slowly breaking down.

As a nurse, it is important to be aware of how you behave toward boy or girl patients. For example, little boys may be reluctant to express fear, especially if they were taught that boys don't cry. Giving children the permission to express their fears while still enabling them to keep their sense of identity can be a difficult but satisfying task.

Sexual Orientation

This third component of sexual identity is sexual identity is related to whom and to which sex the child is attracted. Although sexual orientation may vary throughout the life cycle, it is typically determined in early adolescence. As Kinsey stated in the Kinsey report, at different times during one's life one may have various degrees of attraction to the same or opposite gender.

There has always been tremendous controversy regarding the etiology of homosexuality. As with gender identity, there is no one explanation for why some people are heterosexual, others bisexual, and still others homosexual or gay; there are only numerous theories.

Some theorists believe that homosexuality is caused by biological influences, such as a gene that determines to whom we feel attracted. Other theorists believe that homosexuality is the result of environmental or psychological experiences, perhaps some traumatic event that occurred during childhood, or inadequate love from the mother or father. As a nurse it is important to realize that at least, 10% of the patient population will be exclusively homosexual. This number may be much higher near a large city such as New York, Miami, or San Francisco.

Although sexual orientation begins at an early age, it is usually not expressed until adolescence or beyond. Because of their own sense of *homophobia* (fear of gay people or being gay), some men and women never express their true orientation, or "come out of the closet."

THE SCHOOL-AGE CHILD (6—9 YEARS)

Erikson believed that the tasks of the fourth stage of life were centered around *industry versus inferiority*. At this time children want to engage in the tasks of the real world. They learn cooperation by being involved in peer group activities, and clubs, groups, and even gangs of same-sex children become very important. A sense of mastery at school is an important catalyst for the development of self-esteem. A negative mode of expression frequently experienced at this time is increased confrontational problems with authorities.

Although Freud termed this period of life the *latency period*, this interpretation has been seriously challenged, because there is truly active interest in the other sex at this time. However, this interest is not typically acted upon in the same way that an adult acts out his or her sexuality.

At this stage of development, sexual expression is frequently a same-sex experience. It is also common to share in genital manipulation and exploration with either sex. Although children of this age are curious about their own sexual anatomy, their peers' anatomy, and even their parents' anatomy, they are typically private in terms of overt sexual expression. Sex roles become further differentiated as separation from parents and integration into the world of school occurs.

As nurses we must be aware that at this age children are still very fearful of shots, hospitals, and any kind of invasive procedure. Any illness can threaten the child's emerging sense of self. "Little boys don't cry" and "girls are made of sugar and spice" frequently challenge the child's resources in terms of coping with illness and its possible assault upon body image. Therefore, it is very important to keep lines of communication open not only with the parents but also with the child. This is a threatening time to be in the hospital, and both parents and their children need all of the emotional support possible so that the illness does not become more traumatic than necessary.

Sexual Concerns of Children

As previously stated, being sick, being small, and being in a hospital can make a child fearful, scared, and regressive in behavior. The hospital is also a place where many of the values and behaviors that parents try to encourage in their small children are not only not reinforced but also challenged. Needless to say, this creates a very anxiety-producing situation for not only the child but also for the parents, physician, and nurse.

Nudity

The amount of nudity within the home is dictated by many factors, including cultural mores, the attitude of the parents toward nudity, religious and moral upbringing, and finally the parental relationship. However, it is inevitable that some form of mutual viewing will eventually occur in the home. How that is handled by the parents can give children very strong messages about how they should feel about their own body.

There is nearly a universal curiosity on the part of children about how the unclothed parents' bodies may look. What do mommy and daddy look like without their clothes on? Children with siblings are also curious about their brothers and sisters. However, parents are frequently uncomfortable with nudity and convey this message to their children. Parents do not have to verbally convey disapproval to communicate their feelings: children can perceive their parents' discomfort just by body language and other nonverbal cues.

Nurses, especially those with many years of hospital experience, may eventually become desensitized to nudity. Therefore, it is important to realize that in the hospital nudity may cause great emotional conflict for the child. The frequent need for invasive procedures and urinary catheters and also the necessity for sponge baths, backless gowns, and bedpans all contribute to the child's risk of being exposed. This may cause great anxiety for both the child and the parents.

It is important to be aware of these anxieties. Be matter-of-fact, but also gentle when undressing a child. As discussed, children can pick up negative messages about their bodies from even nonverbal communication. In addition, avoid slang phases, inappropriate adult humor, or any form of criticism.

Sex Education

How are babies made? This universal childhood question is rarely answered with honesty or comfort. Many parents need advice on how to begin implementing sex education with their children. This topic is discussed in the Focus section of the chapter.

Communication and Rituals

Children typically have rituals for toileting, dressing, and other private activities. Since these rituals all contribute to a child's sense of control, maintaining them whenever possible can be very helpful to the child's mental health.

It is also helpful to ask parents and other caregivers the words that they use for sexual organs, elimination, and so on because there is a wide diversity of words used for the genitalia and elimination. Using toys as a vehicle for communication can also be a very nonthreatening way to help children express themselves. Frequently children who are unable to verbalize their anxieties about the rituals of hospitalization can express their feelings through role playing and toys.

Masturbation

This is frequently used by the child to lower anxiety. Since hospitalization is likely to increase anxiety, it is not unusual to see children masturbating more frequently in this often tense environment. Therefore, be aware of your own feelings about masturbation. Although you may be uncomfortable or feel negative about this behavior, it is important to be sensitive to the needs and the self-esteem of children, and not make them feel shameful about masturbation.

Fear of Molestation

This may be a major concern of patients and their families. From infancy, children are typically told about the possibility that "bad" people may someday hurt them. "Good touch, bad touch" is frequently discussed in households. In the hospital situation you may get children who are petrified when an adult goes near their genitalia because they have been taught by their parents that it is wrong to let anyone touch them.

Unfortunately, sexual abuse is common in our culture, with reports stating that as many as one in four children are abused. Therefore, it is also very likely that you may someday care for a child who has been sexually abused. With no clear previous clinical history to rely on, the diagnosis may easily be missed unless all nurses are very alert to this possibility.

Sexually abused children are frequently clinging, weepy, and very frightened when they are cared for by strangers. Suspicious marks or abrasions, unexplained pain when walking, or acting in a sexually inappropriate way are all signs of abuse. Children who have bleeding or unusual discharges from their genitals should also make the nurse suspicious of sexual abuse.

Caring for a hospitalized child is a difficult and frequently traumatic event for the parent, the child, and the nurse. The nurse professional must not only address medical and health issues but must also help maintain the psychosexual integrity of the child. As discussed, these are numerous variables that have to be considered. These include the physical, the psychosocial, and sexual tasks of the growing child. Although universal issues have been presented, it is important to remember that each child is an individual and will bring into the medical situation his or her own unique ways of coping and perceiving the experience. It is the responsibility of the nurse to respect and maintain, as much as possible, the sexual health of the small child.

ABUSE OF CHILDREN

It is important for a nurse to be aware that there are several categories of abuse: physical abuse, neglect, sexual abuse, and emotional abuse. A child may be victim of one or all of these. For a detailed discussion of the impact of abuse on children. See the Focus Topic following.

As nurses we are legally required to report any case of suspected child abuse, whether it is psychological, physical, or sexual abuse. This is an important trust issue for the child and something that you need to be sensitive about when caring for a scared child in a frightening hospital setting. Also be aware of the proper legal protocols for reporting sexual abuse in your state.

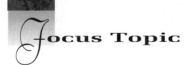

Focus Topic

The Impact of Physical, Emotional, and Sexual Abuse on Children, by Marion E. Rudek, RNC, MSN CRNP

Abusive and violent behavior infiltrates the developing minds of our children like a thin, poisonous vapor cloud. Suspicion must always be present in the minds of all observant lay persons, teachers, health professionals, and neighbors who seek to protect the vulnerability of children. The following situations illustrate various degrees of childhood maltreatment.

An outburst occurs in the middle of the shopping market. A mother turns red with rage upon her 3-year-old because he stalls her movement toward an aisle by picking up a small item near the checkout. She enters into a verbal attack and violently slaps his hands and bottom. He becomes like a rag doll, limp, nonresistant, and whimpering. She drags him by his arm socket. He has bruises on his legs and arms.

A 4-month-old infant is brought to the emergency department with second-degree scalding burns from submersion at bath time. The admitting nurse notices an obvious demarcation line at midtorso with a splash pattern along the right upper extremity. A routine x-ray series points to tiny fractures of the ribs with different stages of healing. Emergency department records are found in two additional nearby health centers.

The school nurse is asked to aid a 9-year-old female student who has fainted. Further evaluation reveals frank hemorrhage on her underwear. Her teacher further voices concern that the student was limping and was unable to sit through her morning class. The girl's affect is unusually glum and listless.

Mrs. A comments to the postman that the 6-year-old boy in the corner lot seems to sit in front of the window for extended periods rocking back and forth. She has never seen him playing outdoors.

Sally is 5 months pregnant. She and her boyfriend open a thin package of white powder and proceed to snort the contents. This is part of a "weekly" ritual, sometimes as frequent as every other day. She is on a cloud in moments; then she crashes and begs for another hit.

The nurse should be aware that abuse and neglect of children span their entire growth cycle, and vary in degree from obvious to hidden. Physical and behavioral indicators are most noticeable; the indicators of emotional neglect are less clear. The progression of events is often centered around a "cycle of violence." Abusers were once themselves abused, and they carry the secret of maltreatment through the generations.

Family dynamics and coping abilities also influence some instances of abuse. For example, a family experiencing a stressful life event may become maladaptive. The tension and outcome of the particular trauma may trigger a pattern of abusive behavior. Addictions to alcohol and drugs may also chemically hinder the mental response and attitude of the caregiver.

Abuse and neglect cross all cultures and economic classes. Although poverty, racism, and gang culture are catalysts for maltreatment, abuse is not partial to poverty and middle-class and wealthy individuals with an abusive nature also exist.

History of Abuse

Infants and children have been connected to sacrificial gestures and maltreatment since biblical times. The murder of first-born, females, imperfects, or disfigured children was practiced up through the 19th century despite a refinement of Church laws in A.D. 438. Industrialization continued abuse through child labor and cruelty. A sensational book written by Charles Dickens, *Oliver Twist*, highlights the constant abuse of children during those years.

The turning point in child abuse awareness came in 1874, when an 8-year-old foundling named Mary Ellen was taken under the protective action of a charity worker, Etta Wheeler. Mary was being battered and assaulted, but no authority would intervene. Mrs. Wheeler turned to the Society for the Prevention of Cruelty to Animals for assistance. She succeeded in gaining imprisonment of the woman offender and orphanage placement for Mary Ellen.

Nearly 250 protective societies for children arose out the care for Mary Ellen. Yet abuse still remained widespread. Although two pediatricians traced radiology findings to suspicion of parental maltreatment in the 1940s the medical field did not mount a strong retaliation to physical abuse in children until the late 1960s.

The first description of the "battered child syndrome" appeared in the *Journal of the American Medical Association (JAMA)* by C. Henry Kempe and Associates in 1962. State laws governing child abuse were developed, and within a year laws were passed encouraging advocacy to diagnose and intervene on behalf of battered children by health professionals. By 1966, child abuse mandates existed throughout the country.

High-Risk Indicators

There are certain physical and behavioral clues that should alert nurses to abuse.

- Physical indicators of abuse span an array of skin and musculoskeletal alterations. Unexplained bruises, welts, burns and blisters, fractures, and open wounds or denuded areas are possible indicators of abuse. In some children each type of skin alteration may be in a different stage of healing. The skin may form clusters or patterns that bear the shapes of inflicting objects (such as rope burn, electric iron, or buckle). Accompanying behaviors may include a shy, withdrawn child, fear of parents or avoidance of the home, and actual statements of physical harm. Children may also become apprehensive or overly aggressive for their developmental age.

- The nurse should realize that physical neglect encompasses basic physiological needs of food, shelter, medical care, and safety. Children who suffer from hunger, poor hygiene, lack of supervision, and inappropriate dress may be victims of abuse. Poor nutrition may contribute to fatigue and lack of alertness. Suspicious actions include stealing, street habitation, prostitution, alcohol or drug use, and notable abandonment of the caregiver.

- Sexual abuse must be carefully assessed in accordance with male and female findings related to maturational growth. For example, deviations from normal hymen diameter and thickness, such as a crescent-shaped, ridged, or thinned hymen, may be present. Bruising of the vaginal and anal areas with torn, bleeding, or unbalanced, worn tissues are definite red flags of forced sexual intercourse. Pain, itching, and presence of semen or sexually transmitted disease are also obvious indicators.

- The range of emotional behaviors that may be exhibited as the result of sexual abuse include withdrawal or promiscuity, fantasy, advanced sexual knowledge, bizarre outbursts, preoccupation with the genitals, or hysteria when private areas are touched during examinations. Running away from home and engaging in delinquent behavior may also indicate that the child had been sexually abused. Pregnancy, especially in an adolescent, is a common finding in families where there is serious dysfunction or incest and rape.

Emotional Abuse

Is the most difficult type of maltreatment to identify and assess in the child. Continued isolation and verbal abuse may result in an array of phobic, neurotic, antisocial, and obsessive habits. A child may withdraw, become overly gregarious or promiscuous, or lag or oversucceed in developmental tasks. Suicide attempts such as through drug overdose may be a cry for help. Hypochondriasis and/or Munchausen syndrome may exist. For example, the parent inflicts physical ailments through artificial means, such as laxative-induced diarrhea that creates the development of these conditions.

The nurse should realize that children who are abused may show depression, social isolation, eating disorders, secretive activity, poor school performance, and regression. Poor self-esteem is another important indicator of emotional abuse.

An Overview of Developmental Ages and Abuse

Fetal Period

There is a large amount of controversy regarding when the fetus is regarded as a separate individual. The conflict over fetal versus maternal rights has complicated the determination of child abuse during the perinatal period. Perinatal abuse may include inattention to prenatal care or nutrition, desire for abortion or miscarriage, substance abuse, or exposure to physical assault.

Significant others play a role in the acceptance and degree of emotional support the mother will receive. The father plays an important supportive role, and influences how the mother will cope with the pregnancy and treat herself and her child. Noncommitted relationships may prevent maternal attachment from developing, and further lack of family or significant support may create ambivalence regarding the task of mothering.

Pregnancy may be planned or unplanned. The unwanted child is an obvious candidate for maltreatment. Early onset of delivery with preterm labor may also affect the bonding of the mother. Newborn illness and/or any resulting permanent handicap increases the risk of stress and tension in the family. Abusive behavior may also develop from anger and chronic fatigue related to caregiving.

The obvious use of alcohol, heroin, marijuana, cocaine, or other substances alone or in combination with one another during pregnancy has growing medical and legal implications. The loss of the infant's life due to the mother's destructive behavior may be viewed as an imposition of wrongful life. In fact there is a growing debate in the legal field over what is known as "intent to harm."

Allegations of child abuse or neglect during the fetal period are currently extending the legal protective rights of children. These efforts are aimed at decreasing immediate perinatal health risks such as seizures, sleep state disorders, cardiac dysrhythmias, placental bleeding, HIV transmission, and sudden infant death syndrome (SIDS).

Infants

The first year of life represents the most rapid period of physical growth. Emotional needs advance to create a balance of trust and dependency. According to Mahler, infants disengage from their symbiotic relationship to the mother but retain a degree of refueling for comfort. Erikson describes the primary developmental task of this age group as trust versus mistrust. In a balanced experience, infants can feel free to explore while developing a sense of self-worth through their caregivers' behaviors.

Early deprivation at the infancy stage contributes to delayed interactive abilities as well as disruption of sleep states and developmental milestones. A listless, apathetic infant who lacks eye contact and has growth and developmental delays demonstrates maltreatment. Failure to thrive can have organic causes such as metabolic deficiencies, but the psychological component is essential for normal responses. Infants who are rejected, or who receive inconsistent care or ambivalence cannot establish trust and will lack the responses needed to fulfill basic dependency needs. They may display withdrawal, irritability, hyper-alertness, anxiety, and avoidance. They will learn to turn within and away from the insecure environment.

Young Children

Toddlerhood through school age represents vast growth of cognition and independence. Once children separate from parents, they can master a wide range of skills with assurance and safe guidance from the parent.

Progressive autonomy is achieved once young children increase their mobility with walking. Verbal skills expand and allow them to express specific needs. However, these needs are self-centered, and parents may become confused because children frequently pay close attention to them in one moment and avoid them in the next. A misinterpretation of this immature behavior may frustrate parents and initiate a cycle of maltreatment.

Preschoolers have more sophisticated language but remain self-absorbed. The development of initiative and peer relationships extends their interactive sphere. During this period, however, parents are still the markers of what is right or wrong, and young children may internalize blame and therefore have lower self-esteem if not treated with understanding.

School-age Children

These children have the advantage of extended relationships within groups and additional exposure to authority through teachers and other adults. Competence and more developed cognition give them better insight. Maltreatment during this young age span may result in the obvious display of developmental delays, speech impediments and lags in social skills. Depression and withdrawal are one end of the reactive spectrum, and aggression and anxiety are the other. Negative self-concept may be a symptom in any child who has sleeping and eating disturbances, agitation, and/or acting-out behavior.

Management of the clinical condition of the child is complex, and even more difficult if the maltreatment has extended over a longer period of childhood. All maturational points in the development of the young child involve adult models, especially the parents, but an abusive parent will not have the insight or resources to see and correct the reaction and behavior which the abused or maltreated child displays.

Adolescents

Pubescence and adolescence incorporate earlier learning while moving toward independence. In this stage children have greater opportunities to expand relationships that will either resolve prior difficulties or reinforce earlier patterns.

Preteens and teenagers must also adjust to the complexity of sexual development. This stage is the second most rapid stage in terms of growth over a short period of time. Behaviors become potentially more lethal at this age because the individual is more cognitively aware of a variety of coping strategies to deal with the ongoing struggle for maturity and peer acceptance. In this struggle the adolescent is more apt to engage in destructive behavior. For example, any aggressive behavior may lead adolescents to express themselves through drug abuse and alcohol dependency. Sexual curiosity may lead them to sexual experimentation without regard for protection against sexually transmitted disease or pregnancy.

These drastic changes may also be the turning point for a parent-child relationship that was stable in the younger years. The physical maturity and sexual development of a young girl or boy may be the impetus for channeling maltreatment toward sexual abuse. For example, a father may suddenly realize that his daughter has significant breast development and is coming of age for sexual expression. Former verbal abuse may then be channeled into sexual abuse.

A prolonged experience of maltreatment may manifest itself in obvious psychiatric illness. Repeated loss of control may result in several different categories of illness, including attention deficit disorder, chronic depression, anxiety, and separation problems. Child maltreatment that has reached the point of constant exposure also has the risk of accommodation: that is, lifelong acceptance of abuse requires the child to adapt. Such a child will learn to accept the rules that have been established by the abuser and may not actively seek to run away from the situation. Accommodation signifies internalized self-blame. The child feels that he or she is not deserving of a different situation or cannot perceive how the abuse is unhealthy. Sexually abused children may integrate the relationship with the parent as normal in order to emotionally survive.

The sexual abuse victim also encounters the experience of shame. The abuser may convince the child that he or she provokes the situation. These beliefs hinder the ability of the child to safely disclose the abuser. This secrecy endangers the future development of close relationships, and lack of power and control creates a stigma toward sexuality. Sexual dysfunction and social isolation are highly probable in a continuing situation of sexual adult and/or incest.

Abused Children as Adults

The nurse must realize that victimization as a child does not vanish from the psyche. Positive interventions will improve the coping abilities of the adult; however, it is unclear if the scars from the prior maltreatment do truly heal. Research has been able to link prior maltreatment to lasting social, psychological, and intellectual deficits in adulthood.

Child abuse is a form of trauma. There has been found to be a striking trend of post-traumatic stress syndrome in adults with documented behavioral problems, many of which have been currently associated with child abuse. For example, the victims continue to have a higher rate of sexual assault toward children when they themselves become adults.

Adults who have reported sexual abuse as children also appear more likely to suffer from chronic depression, suicide attempts, eating disorders, and general anxiety. These adult disorders seem to derive from an underlying insult to self-esteem.

Positive Interventions

Research has suggested that although the abused child has a greater chance of becoming an abuser in later life, the bleak cycle of victimization can be broken. Abused children who receive interventions have a better chance of improving their self-esteem and capacity for close relationships. One significant role model can soften the experience and help recreate a warm and caring environment.

The key to prevention is to recognize the physical and behavioral signs of abuse in the child. Instinct may also suggest looking into a pattern of troubled family interaction. The earlier the intervention occurs in the development of the child, the greater the child's chance of achieving more normal emotional and sexual functioning as an adult. Nurses need to be aware that physical, emotional, and sexual abuse can be identified, halted, and treated. They can make a significant lifelong positive difference.

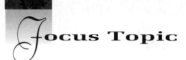

Focus Topic

Sex Education for Children

Parents do not really have a choice as to whether their children will learn about sex. Children learn about sexuality from the overt and covert messages that their parents, their friends, other adults, and the media give them. These include messages about gender role, relationships, sexual behavior, nudity, and masturbation. However, parents do have a choice as to whether or not they will participate in a verbal, straightforward, open manner in their children's sex education.

By interacting with their children, parents can give them the message that sex is something that can be discussed, that it is not taboo. This interaction can also give children the skills they need to communicate both negative and pleasurable messages that they have received or experienced regarding their evolving sexuality.

One of the most uncomfortable topics for adults and parents is coming to terms with their children's sexuality. As a consequence, one of the most uncomfortable topics for children is coming to terms with not only their own sexuality but their parents' sexuality. Frequently a perpetual cycle of discomfort and ignorance evolves between children and their parents.

However, adult values can typically only be modified, whereas young children's values can still be shaped and developed. Therefore, it is very advantageous to begin early sex education, before discomfort occurs. The following are guidelines that you can give parents regarding practical and helpful pointers when talking to their young children about sex.

1. When you discuss sex with young children, try to speak in a comfortable and matter-of-fact manner. Be as spontaneous as possible so that the child will role-model your behavior and become more comfortable talking about sex.

2. Don't lecture about sex. Communication needs to be two-way. Young children cannot typically concentrate for more than very short periods of time. The questions that are not answered in one session can always be readdressed at another time. Introduce single concepts during a session so that the child does not become overwhelmed.

3. Be a role model. Sex education is more than biology: it encompasses feelings, attitudes, and good decision-making skills. Encourage your children to be comfortable in talking about feelings. They can learn about healthy intimacy from your behavior.

4. Be aware that children will typically "tune out" inappropriate age-related material. Either it will go over their heads or they will just not relate to it.

5. Use correct terminology for body parts. Most children know universal words for all body parts other than the genitals. Omitting these words or giving them baby names is giving your child the message that perhaps these words are dirty. Why else wouldn't mommy or daddy say them? Learning correct terminology will also enable them to better communicate with you if another adult has gone beyond appropriate boundaries with them.

6. Children love to mimic. They are also great nonverbal readers. If small children say a dirty word, explain to them calmly why they shouldn't say the word. With small children such explanations as "Other people may get upset if they hear those words" may be helpful.

7. Small children need to know how to protect themselves from sexual abuse. You need to let them know that it is okay to say no to an adult.

8. You don't need to be a sex education expert. If you don't have the answer to a question, that's okay. Look it up, call your doctor, or ask a valued friend about it.

9. Reinforce your teaching. Come back to the topic often so that you can clear up any misconceptions and reinforce old and new learning.

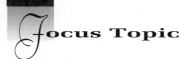

ocus Topic

An Overview of Childhood

The theories that are overviewed in this chapter include Erik Erikson's Eight Stages of Life, Object-relations theory, and Sigmund Freud and psychosexual development. Family life cycle concerns as well as human sexuality issues for the child are overviewed, including stressors frequently experienced in the hospital setting. However, it is important to recognize that because each child is unique, the developmental timing of these stages varies, and therefore the following is only a broad guideline.

There are seven childhood developmental stages:

Prenatal: conception to birth

Infancy: birth through 1 year

Toddler: 1 to 4 years

Preschool: 4 to 6 years

School-age: 6 to 9 years

Preadolescent: 9 to 12 years

Adolescent: 12 through 21 years

Refer to Table 3-1 for an overview of the first six developmental stages. Chapter 4 discusses adolescence.

Table 3-1
Developmental Stages During Childhood

Birth Through 1 Year

Object-relations theory:

Autistic period: Newborn infants have no sense that their body has boundaries or that there are other people within the world.

- Outside stimuli have no effect.

- Respond only to their own physiological needs.

- Stimuli of mother draws them into the world.

Symbiotic phase: till 1 year

- Maintain homeostasis (sense of balance in the world).

- Distinguish good and bad experiences.

- Cannot distinguish boundaries.

- Social smile develops with awareness of mother.

Separation Differentiation: till 1 year

- Special bond to mother: 4–5 months

- Body awareness.

- Increasing differentiation: 6 months.

- Checks back as they begin to toddle: 7–8 months (called "practicing").

- Stranger anxiety: compare mother's face to others.

If separation occurs too early, the child may experience a great amount of anxiety.

Freud/oral stage: The mouth is the center of pleasure, and intake of food is pleasurable. The mouth can also be linked to aggression.

Infant is mostly id.

Ego slowly begins to develop with cognition.

Erikson/trust versus mistrust: The infant begins to develop a sense of safety in the world. This is accomplished through good mothering. (The mother does not have to be the biological mother but must be capable of meeting the infant's needs.)

Stage in family life cycle: child-bearing.

Sexuality: Sense of touch is developed through hugging and being held. Sexuality is nongenitally focused, although infants have sexual reactions to stimuli of genitals and other erogenous zones; males may have early masturbation: Gender role conditioning begins.

Stressors related to illness: If children do not have positive physical contact, they may become very anxious, retarded, or autistic. They may develop a lack of sense of safety. If mother is nursing, this experience may be interrupted if child is hospitalized.

Toddler: 1 to 4 years

Object-relations theory: Continued separation from mother and individuation.

- Magical omnipotence.

- Externally supported self-esteem.

- Sense of separateness, gender, beginning autonomy from mother or primary caregiver.

- Self-soothing via recontact and evocative memory with mother.

Freud/anal stage: Develop mastery of own impulses. Major frustration is toilet training: enjoys smearing, playing with feces. First real demand by caregivers to conform.

- Beginning development of ego.

- Learning to hold on and let go.

- Rigidity, only one right way: "mine."

- Perfectionism: collecting, hoarding, resentment of authority. Lacking in self-confidence. Techniques and attitudes of mother important in helping children give up narcissistic omnipotence.

Erikson: autonomy versus shame, doubt. Children need graded independence as they learn to separate successfully from their parents.

They need to develop a sense of self-reliance, adequacy, and mastery. Begin to learn "right" and "wrong." Learn to delay satisfaction for future reward. Begin to learn the process of decision making.

Sexuality: Gender identity: children know that they are either boys or girls. Sex role development: children begin to copy behavior of appropriate sex. Masturbation: guilt and shame occur over one's body if negative messages are received.

Stressors related to illness: Separation from parents. Invasive procedures create a sense of shame. Regression in terms of toilet training and self-care behavior may occur if child is hospitalized. Lack of sense of control. Fear. Separation from family and from daily rituals. May experience bad dreams and/or night terrors. Not always able to draw from previous experiences. Immobilization does not allow child to exercise body and continue physical mastery.

Preschool: 4 to 6 years

Freud/phallic stage, 4th year: Early pregenital stage of sexuality. Attitudes formed during this period are crucial for later heterosexual fulfillment and good relationships with people. Freud developed the following concepts:

Love object is mother.

Oedipus complex: Rivalry with father for possession of mother. Doomed to failure: resolution necessary

Electra Complex: Little girl must change her loyalty love from father to mother and begin to identify with mother.

Castration fear: Partly fear of loss of love of father; fear of castration.

Identification: Learning of sex roles: boys with fathers and girls with mothers.

Superego: Develops more strongly because of incorporation of attitudes of parents. Begins to develop a conscience.

Erikson/initiative versus guilt: Children learn about world and other people. Must learn to assert self without guilt. Imitate parents, engage in cooperate play, enjoy ritualized games. Social conscience emerges. Need experience in decision making. Problems may occur if role model is poor. Fear of loss of parental love can cause anxiety.

- Imitate activities.

- Attention span increases.

- Cooperative play increases.

- Enjoy ritualized games.

- Social conscience emerges.

Stage in family life cycle: childbearing family.

Sexuality: Completion of sex role conditioning; beginning of genital orientation and interest. Masturbation continues. Children may be very curious regarding the genitals of the other sex. They enjoy playing house or doctor.

Stressors related to illness: Separation from parents. Invasive procedures create a sense of shame. Regression in terms of toilet training and self-care behavior. Lack of sense of control, fear and shame. Separation from family and from daily rituals. Bad dreams and sometimes inability to draw from previous experiences. Immobilization does not allow child to exercise body and continue physical mastery.

School age: 6 to 9 years

Object-relations theory: Peers and teachers influence self-concept. Highly differentiated self and object representations.

Freud/latency period: This is widely disputed. We now believe that although children are not typically genitally focused they are still very interested in sexuality.

Industry versus inferiority: Basic modality is to make things and to put things together: completion of a task. Focus is on mastery of tasks. Activities are mainly sex-segregated. Play begins to merge with reality: school is very important in the development of a positive self-concept.

Stage in family life cycle: school-age and small children; child-focused family.

Sexuality: Genital orientation and interest, latency period. Oedipal stage still ongoing (romantic attachment to opposite-sex parent). Children may still play house or doctor.

This is the most vulnerable age for nonsexual experiences to be perceived as genitally arousing. Therefore, we need to be extremely sensitive regarding any invasive procedures and the meaning and interpretation of that experience for the child.

Stressors related to illness: Fear of invasion of body, embarrassment, nudity and shame issues, regression, increased dependency on parents and possibly other siblings, separation from friends, inability to be physically active, loss of school or sport time.

Preadolescence: 9 to 12 years

Object-relations theory: Peers, teachers, and sports stars are very important role models. At this stage the child is a highly differentiated person. Most common age to develop a inferiority complex.

Freud: Still considers this to be period of quiescence. Child will use sublimation, rationalization, and isolation as coping mechanisms.

Stage in family life cycle: There may be children at many different developmental stages within the family. Still a very child-focused family.

Sexuality: Active interest in other sex, basic relationships with own sex. Rather common to share in genital manipulation and exploration with either sex. Pathology relevant to sexual erotic behaviors begins to manifest itself. Prepubescent secondary sex changes begin to occur.

Stressors related to illness: Threats to body image, regression, forced dependence on parents and other adults, embarrassment, fear of illness, separation from family, friends, and familiar routine, absence from school, fear of being infantilized.

BIBLIOGRAPHY

Besharov, D.J. Mandatory reporting of child abuse and research on the effects of prenatal drug exposure. *NIDA Research Monograph,* 1992, 117, 366–384.

Black, C. A., & DeBlassie, R. R. Sexual abuse in male children and adolescents: Indicators, effects, and treatments. *Adolescence*, 1993, 28(109), 123–133.

Cousins, N. *Anatomy of an illness.* New York: Norton, 1979.

Doob, D. Female sexual abuse survivors as patients: Avoiding retraumatization. *Archives of Psychiatric Nursing*, 1992, 6(4), 245–251.

Fry, R. Adult physical illness and childhood sexual abuse. *Journal of Psychosomatic Research*, 1993, 37(2), 89–103.

Ginsburg, H., Wright, L. S., Harrell, P., & Hill, D. W. Childhood victimization: Desensitization effects in the later lifespan. *Child Psychiatry and Human Development*, 1989, 20(1), 59–71.

Goldson, E. The affective and cognitive sequelae of child maltreatment. *Pediatric Clinics of North America*, 1991, 38(6), 1481–1496.

Herman-Staab, B. Antecedents to nonorganic failure to thrive. *Pediatric Nursing*, 1992, 18(6), 579–583.

Hetherington, E. M., & Ross, D. P. *Contemporary readings in child psychology*, (2nd ed.). New York: McGraw-Hill, 1981.

Hyden, P. W., & Gallagher, T. A. Child abuse in the emergency room. *Pediatric Clinics of North America*, 1992, 39(5), 1053–1081.

Irons, T. G. Documenting sexual abuse of a child. *Emergency Medicine*, April 1993, pp. 57–74.

Jurgrau, A. How to spot child abuse. *RN*, October 1990, pp. 26–32.

Klaus, M. H., Leger, T., & Trause, M. A. *Maternal attachment and mothering disorders* (2nd ed.). Johnson & Johnson Baby Products, 1982.

Law, J., & Conway, J. Effect of abuse and neglect on the development of children's speech and language. *Developmental Medicine and Child Neurology*, 1992, 34(11), 943–948.

Leventhal, J. M., Horowitz, S. M., Rude, C., & Stier, D. M. Maltreatment of children born to teenage mothers: A comparison between the 1960's and 1980's. *Journal of Pediatrics*, 1993, 122(2), 314–319.

Mahler, M. S., Bergman, A., & Pine, F. *The psychological birth of the human infant: Symbiosis and individuation*. New York: Basic Books, 1975.

Martin, J. A., & Elmer, E. Battered children grown up: A follow-up study of individuals severely maltreated as children. *Child Abuse and Neglect*, 1992, 16(1), 75–87.

McGuire, T. L., & Feldman, K. W. Psychologic morbidity of children subjected to Munchausen syndrome by proxy. *Pediatrics*, 1989, 83(2), 289–292.

Shengold, L. *Soul murder: The effects of childhood abuse and deprivation*. New York: Fawcett Columbine, 1989.

Showers, S. Shaken baby syndrome: The problem and a model for prevention. *Child Today*, 1992, 21(2), 34–37.

Chapter 4

The Countdown Toward Adulthood: Adolescence and the Teenage Years

Only the day before, Sara was outside playing tag with two of her friends. That evening she had sat and watched television with her parents. School had been fun that day as they prepared for the Halloween party. Now Sara was crying in her room. She had just gone to the bathroom and her panties were stained with blood. She was scared. Could she be bleeding because she had hurt herself or did it mean that she was sick? Or could it be her period? Her girl-friends referred to this bleeding as their "friend." She was too scared to ask.

It was 1 A.M. in the morning and Mark was waiting for everyone to go to sleep. Why didn't they hurry up. For the third time in 2 weeks he had woken up with his pajamas wet. He was horrified! What if his mother or younger brother found out? Could he be wetting his bed? Was he terribly sick? How could he find out? In the meantime as soon as the house was quiet he would go down and wash his pajamas.

Sexuality, in the genital sense of the term, has its onset at puberty. Adolescence may be experienced as not only one of the most exciting periods of life but also a time of great difficulty and conflict. That is because adolescents must successfully adjust to enormous physical and mental changes. They will typically enter adolescence as children and leave this period as almost adults.

PSYCHOSOCIAL TASKS OF ADOLESCENCE

Erikson termed the maturational crisis of adolescence the need to resolve the issue of *identity versus identity confusion.* During this fifth stage of psychosocial development Erikson believed that adolescents must successfully develop a clear concept of their identity. They must also begin to consider what role they will eventually take in our society.

This decision-making process is shaped by both parental and peer group expectations. Identity is also influenced by the cultural values of his the adolescent's peer group world. Peer group values may be the most powerful motivator. For example, being a popular football player or school cheerleader may be a primary goal.

Adolescence is also a period of rapid physical changes which necessi-tate new body image perceptions. The little girl will begin to become a woman, and the little boy will begin to become a man. Initially, these changes can be very threatening, and significant coping adaptations may be necessary to adjust to them.

In both males and females an underlying cause of anxiety is the need to be similar to one's peers. Obviously however, these concerns are different for each sex. For example, the young adolescent girl may worry about the size and shape of her breasts. She may also worry that she is too tall or too awkward. Other newly developing secondary sex characteristics such as pubic hair and widening hips may also cause her anxiety. The adolescent boy is frequently concerned about the size and even shape of his penis. He may worry that he is too short or not as strong as some of his peers. He may wonder if he should take steroids so that he can become stronger than the other boys. As his voice deepens, he may fear that he may suddenly "squeak" out an answer in class.

PSYCHOSEXUAL DEVELOPMENTAL STAGES

The physical changes of adolescence occur along a time continuum which is divided into three stages: early, middle, and late adolescence.

Early Adolescence

Early adolescence typically occurs between the ages of 11 to 14. This stage is characterized by concern about physical changes. Ambivalence regarding independence versus protection from parents and from other adults in authority is also common. Early adolescence is also characterized by egocentricity, the belief that the needs of the individual exist before those of anyone else.

Finally, during this early stage adolescents need to begin a dramatic separation from their family of origin and develop a unique, independent sense of identity. Some developmental theorists have defined this period of time as the second separation from parents. The first separation, as discussed in the prior chapter, was during very early childhood.

During this time, adolescents also begin to challenge not only their own beliefs but most of their parents' beliefs as well. Therefore this can be a time torn with strife. There is frequent unease and conflict between adolescents and their parents as separation is negotiated. No longer is the child's world a safe haven, and no longer are the parents the unchallenged authorities. The adolescent frequently perceives even trivial issues as catastrophic.

Parents also have a developmental task to accomplish. It is their task to allow this separation to occur. As they struggle to let go of the control they believed they had over their children many parents find this a troubling and frightening time. No longer can they keep their children safe. Now they must have faith that their adolescents are capable of making good decisions regarding drugs, alcohol, driving, and sexuality. In addition, parents are also struggling with their own challenges in self-perception and body image. Many are coping with the developmental tasks of entering middle age and are experiencing the losses characteristic of that period.

As nurses it is important to understand why adolescents test their parents to such an extreme and why for many parents this is such a troubling time. Perhaps the motivation behind the adolescent's behavior is to make life so conflictual for the parents that they are finally able and willing to let go of their child and allow him or her to enter the world. They must accept the loss of their power and control over their child. Through all of this the nurse can act as both a confidant and counselor for many troubled teens and confused parents.

Nurses should also be aware that young adolescents have certain concerns about body image. Physical growth may be perceived as too fast or too slow. Genital hair, body hair, and breast appearance may not be pleasing. Other reactions and concerns include curiosity and concern about the normalcy of their bodies. Newly emerging sexual feelings and the behavior of themselves and their peers can also create anxiety. The nurse can be a safe and trustworthy adult for the teen to confide their concerns.

Some therapists and counselors believe that adolescents who are sexually promiscuous usually come from families that have significant psychosocial dysfunction; that is, the parents have very poor relationships and destructive behaviors between themselves or with their children. Frequently there is sexual abuse, promiscuity, or alcoholism within the home.

Sexual activity in adolescents may be symbolically expressive of the need to have control over their lives. It may also be used as an attempt to have their parents pay attention to them. Frequently it is not sex that these young adolescents are seeking but stability and love. Therefore, nurses and other health professionals need to be aware of the underlying dynamics of the young adolescent. All too frequently these adolescents fall under our care because they are pregnant or need birth control information. We need to not only address the physical components of their care but also consider the underlying dynamics of why these teens are choosing to be sexual at such an early age.

It is within the scope of our nursing practice to address developmental issues, to offer counseling, and to present psychoeducational programming. It is the author's opinion that frequently the adolescent is not really presenting for the "pill" but for a hug. These are important issues to keep in mind as we create a balanced plan of psychosexual care.

Middle Adolescence

Middle adolescence occurs between the ages of 14 and 17. The most significant concern at this age is the need for peer approval. Frequently, there is a desire to separate from old friends and create a set of new peer group friends who share the same values and attitudes. Choosing new friends may sometimes be confusing because adolescents may still be struggling with their own emerging values.

The nurse must recognize that these adolescents frequently experiment with risk-taking behavior. This may be expressed by risky sexual behavior and alcohol or drug abuse. This age group is quickly becoming one of the highest risk groups for AIDS, which is a major concern for health professionals, teens, and their parents. Nurses need to take a lead in giving accurate AIDS education.

Peer group behavior also strongly encourages or discourages sexual activity. Like younger adolescents, adolescents who have sexual intercourse at this age frequently do so to prove themselves and/or to feel loved and accepted. Rarely during this developmental stage are concerns regarding commitment, preferences about sexual pleasuring, or even contraception discussed prior to sexual intercourse. Teenagers are not typically comfortable discussing sexuality with anyone, especially their parents.

Therapeutic interventions for these concerns include peer group counseling and sex education books that are written with the culture and developmental level of the teen in mind. Other useful interventions include providing privacy when discussing sexuality with teenage patients and trying to provide a nonjudgmental atmosphere. It may be difficult for nurses to cope with their own concern for these teenagers, yet they need to remain professionally objective so that they can be effective in enabling teenagers to trust and bond with them.

Late Adolescence

Late adolescence is typically defined as the ages between 17 and 21. It is assumed that at this stage of life the teenager has become more cognitively mature, and for the majority of teenagers this may well be true. The development of healthy intimacy and the need for and experience of long-term relationships may occur. The presence of a strong moral and value system should have also developed. Further exploration regarding sexual identity and orientation may still be occurring.

Becoming intellectually competent after high school is also an important accomplishment. Developing a vocation that will make adolescents self-sufficient is a necessary task of this period of life. Without the freedom of financial independence and autonomy it is difficult not only to separate from one's family of origin but also to maintain a strong and healthy sense of self-esteem.

Another task of late adolescence is the need and frequently the courage to separate from old peer groups. Young adults often develop a new group of friends that have compatible social and moral values. This new group may frequently be different from the cultural and socioeconomic world in which they were raised.

As discussed, it is important for the nurse to remember that teenagers do not exist in a timeless vacuum, and that for many parents their children's adolescence is occurring as they are also beginning to confront their own midlife issues. The emerging sexuality of a teenage daughter or son may feel threatening and uncomfortable to a parent who is working through his or her issues regarding changing body image, menopause, and declining sexual activity.

Together these developmental tasks can feel like an overwhelming emotional situation for the family. There may also be grandparents who are confronting medical, financial, and existential issues related to the meaning of their own lives. They are frequently confused by modern teenage behavior and yearn for the "good old days."

Another issue related to separation and individuation is the challenge to family loyalty as adolescents leave the care and perhaps even the value system of their parents. Parents may feel sad and threatened as they see their sons and daughters not totally embrace the values that they believe to be important and that they grew up with, such as going to church every Sunday, working after school, entering the military, or generally following in their parents "footsteps."

A poignantly striking example of this conflict is the parent whose child chooses a bisexual or gay orientation. Working through these conflictual issues and the feelings that they raise for both the parents and the young adult can be traumatic and threatening for the health of the family.

Again, our heightened awareness of these issues will enhance our caregiving in addressing the physical, psychological, and spiritual needs of our patients and their families.

BIOLOGICAL CHANGES

This section of the chapter will present a brief overview of the dramatic physical changes that occur during puberty. This maturational period may take anywhere from 1 1/2 to 6 years to conclude. During this time the adolescent has a tremendous growth spurt and develops the secondary sex characteristics needed for sexual maturation. Girls begin to menstruate, usually around 12.8 years, and boys will develop the ability to ejaculate. By the conclusion of adolescence fertility is established for the majority of boys and girls.

Both males and females have the same hormones. However, these hormones are present in different amounts and trigger different changes in the male and female body. The physical changes that characterize puberty occur as the result of hormonal stimulation. The pituitary gland (the master gland) is responsible for the regulation of these hormonal changes. It is a pea-sized structure located at the base of the brain. The pituitary is divided into the posterior pituitary gland, which is attached to the brain by nerves, and the anterior pituitary gland, which is attached to the brain by blood vessels.

The *anterior pituitary gland* controls the functioning of the ovaries and testes through stimulating hormones it produces called *trophic* (from the Latin "to nourish") *hormones*, or *gonadotropins*. These hormones stimulate the ovaries and testes to secrete the end-product hormones *estrogen*, *progesterone* and *testosterone*.

In the female, the gonadotropins are called *follicle-stimulating hormone (FSH)* and *luteinizing hormone (LH)*. FSH causes the growth of ovarian follicles. As a result of this hormonal stimulation the follicles will release one egg per month during the menstrual cycle. LH triggers ovulation. In the male FSH initiates sperm production and LH stimulates androgen production (see following Figure 4–1) and helps maintain spermatogenesis.

Amazingly, a female baby is born with 500,000 follicles in her ovaries. One follicle will develop monthly into the egg that may eventually join with male sperm to create an embryo. It is important to realize that a biological clock is "ticking" for every female because as she ages her 500,000 follicles are also aging. This accounts for the higher incidence of babies born with Down's syndrome and birth defects to older mothers.

Boys begin to secrete massive amounts of testosterone from the testes and the adrenals. Testosterone, considered to be the main male sex hormone, is responsible for almost all of the physical changes that occur during male puberty. These changes include the development of the male secondary sex characteristics, such as the growth of the penis and testicles and the growth of pubic hair. Males also develop a deeper voice and greater body mass and strength. The presence not only of ejaculatory fluid but also of semen makes them fertile. In contrast to the biological clock that characterizes women's fertility, men are constantly producing new sperm throughout the life cycle.

Physical changes in the girl occur as the result of estrogen which is secreted by the ovaries. The secretion of large amounts of estrogen is responsible for enlarged breast development and the development of feminine body contours, including wider hips and fat deposits in the breasts, hips, and buttocks. Estrogen also produces the growth and maturation of the vagina, uterus, fallopian tubes, and labia minora. Girls at this time become fertile.

For a review of biological changes, see Figure 4-1.

DEVELOPMENTAL PROBLEMS

The following are some of the areas of sexual concern for the adolescent. Both psychosexual and physiological problems frequently need to be addressed and processed by the nurse.

Psychosexual Concerns

Image Disturbances

These are common during this age. As discussed at the beginning of the chapter, adolescents are very concerned about whether their body shapes are normal, or similar to their peers. Every culture has its own unique definition of attractiveness. The culturally defined American, white middle-class ideal for girls is often a "Barbie Doll" image of being slim, blond, and big-breasted. For the male, the ideal cultural image is similar to that of Ken, Barbie's boyfriend. Ken is handsome,

FIGURE 4-1
Effects of Sex Hormones on Pubertal Development

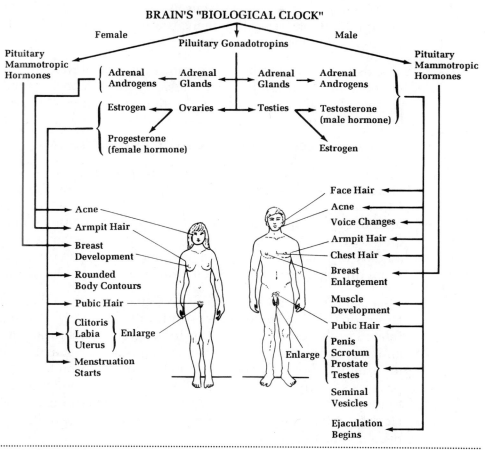

Credit: From John H. Gagnon, *Human Sexuality*, 1977 Glenview, Il: Scott Forseman and Co. ©1977 by John H. Gagnon. Reprinted by permission.

tall, and muscular. The boy who feels he is too short or the girl who, according to our standards, is just too tall may see this as a crisis of tremendous proportions.

Lack of Accurate Information

Lack of information for many adolescents leads to misperceptions and shame. Because adolescence is a period of tremendous anxiety, as nurses we need to refocus some of these tense emotions through education and supportive interest in helping adolescents clarify and discuss their concerns.

For example, it may be helpful to discuss with both mother and daughter the beginning of menstruation. Because mothers frequently influence their daughters' perception of this event, it may be advantageous to help dispel some of the secrecy, myths, and anxieties that both of them may be feeling by discussing the changes that they can expect to happen. Books regarding menstruation for the young girl may also be useful for mother and daughter.

It is also important to be aware and respectful of the culture of your patients and their families. In some cultures the onset of menstruation is viewed with a great amount of religious significance and celebration. In other cultures it is not as acknowledged and even ignored.

Lack of Control Over One's Body

This is another source of anxiety. Suddenly getting one's period in class can be embarrassing for the young girl. Spontaneous erections and wet dreams can cause the young boy anxiety. At this age, erections tend to occur haphazardly and at inappropriate times. They are frequently unrelated to genital sensation and may even be triggered by anxiety or fear. For example, a boy who is called to the front of the room during class may develop a full erection that he cannot hide.

This is an important time of life for fathers to talk to their sons. Unfortunately, for many fathers and sons there may be discomfort related to this conversation. If prior conversations regarding feelings and events have never occurred, communication may now be difficult to initiate. Moreover, many fathers have never been taught how to process sensitive issues, especially since we infrequently teach men the skills of being expressive and comfortable talking to their children. Hopefully this will change as sex education and parenting classes become more common.

The young boy may be frightened and embarrassed by the rapid and seemingly uncontrollable changes that are happening to his body. Along with the normal physical changes that occur, it is also important to help fathers discuss with their sons responsible sexual decision making, contraception, and sexually transmitted diseases.

As nurses we can be role models and resources for communication. If there is no father available, we should be creative in eliciting the help and aid of other willing males who may be willing to work with the adolescent. An example of one such non-profit group is the Big Brothers/Big Sisters Association.

Needless to say, there are multiple biological issues that can cause great distress and anxiety not only for adolescents but also for parents. Although many of these conditions are normal, they can still cause emotional distress. We can help dispel some of that anxiety just by giving these families permission to discuss these issues.

Homosexual Experiences

These are another concern of teenagers as they struggle for identity and comfort in their sexual orientation. Teenagers are in a state of emotional flux and alternate life-styles are commonly tried. Those who find that they are gay usually receive very little support and guidance, and frequently they feel a tremendous amount of shame and guilt. The AIDS crisis has made this an even more lonely experience.

Sexual Disinterest

The sexually uninterested adolescent may also feel uncomfortable and different. There are many reasons why teenagers may feel sexually uninterested, including the wish to delay growing up or to deny authority. Some teenagers are also fearful of themselves and their sexuality.

Physiological Concerns

Pain and Discomfort

Discomfort related to normal physiological changes may occur. *Dysmenorrhea*, which is a spasmodic cramping of the uterus, frequently begins with the development of ovulatory periods. These painful periods typically occur around 15 years of age. Dysmenorrhea can also be characterized by backache, headache, a feeling of being bloated, and sometimes even diarrhea, nausea, or vomiting.

It is theorized that dysmenorrhea occurs as the result of increased prostaglandins from the endometrium (lining of the uterus). This condition is called *primary dysmenorrhea* because it occurs without the presence of any pelvic abnormality. Dysmenorrhea peaks at approximately age 18, and the frequency of primary dysmenorrhea usually diminishes by the mid-20s. Secondary dysmenorrhea is diagnosed when a specific pelvic abnormality is found in the presence of the same symptoms.

Another influence on the perception of pain is related to the messages that the young girl gets from her mother, her sisters, her peers, and her culture. For example, if she is part of a family of women who experience a great amount of pain during menstruation or view menstruation as "dirty" or burdensome, she may well anticipate the pain and wait for it to occur.

When these anxieties occur, visual aids and books can be helpful in dispelling false and misleading information. A relaxed tone of voice and general easiness with these subjects will help you role-model lack of fear.

Other Problems

Secondary amenorrhea and delayed sexual maturation related to delayed menarche are also concerns for girls. *Secondary amenorrhea* is the absence of menses after there have been normal periods for at least 1 year; *delayed menarche* means that the girl has never menstruated. For both of these menstrual conditions it is important for the nurse to take a careful medical history. They can be a source of major concern for the young girl and her family.

Secondary amenorrhea may be a symptom of anorexia. Eating disorders have now reached epidemic proportions in adolescent girls. Nurses need to be aware of the symptomatology that highlights this very serious disorder. Some of these symptoms include weight loss, amenorrhea, hair loss, apathy, increased exercise and increased "interest" in feeding others.

When sexual maturation is delayed, boys also have an array of worries and concerns. One concern related to delayed adolescence occurs when the boy is the shortest in his class; usually because of a delay of his growth spurt. Sometimes these conditions are caused by gonadal or pituitary disease. Genetics can also play an important role in height. Weight, small penis size, and even the advent of acne can cause severe anxiety.

EXPERIENCING SEXUAL BEHAVIOR

Normal sexual activity can be a catalyst or a reaction to everyday stressors. Although adolescents can find sex pleasurable, they frequently have feelings of shame, guilt, and anxiety when coping with their emerging sexuality. These feelings can be manifested behaviorally and emotionally. There is a whole range of sexual activity that may be experienced by the teenager. The following discussion covers some of those activities.

Premarital Sex

Premarital heterosexual activity is common in contemporary American culture. Researchers estimate that as many as 50 to 60% of teenage girls and 70 to 75% of adolescent boys will have intercourse before the age of 18. Increasingly, teenagers as young as 11 years of age are becoming sexual.

The incidence of teenage pregnancy has increased dramatically over the past two decades in the United States. Some estimate that as many as 1.1 million women under the age of 20 will get pregnant annually, and a staggering 50% of those 1.1 million teenage pregnancies end in miscarriage or abortion. Sadly, 40% of teenagers who leave high school because of pregnancy never return to get a high school diploma. These unwed mothers have to make many difficult decisions in a short period of time regarding abortion, adoption, marriage, and single parenthood.

Sex is frequently used as a rebellion or a means of separation from parents. No longer children, but not yet adults, teenagers struggle to successfully separate from their parents. Paradoxically, as a result, they frequently become parents themselves.

Early intercourse may also trigger unsatisfying sexual experiences that may well set up future patterns for repeated unsatisfying relationships through adulthood. The cost to self-esteem can also be traumatic if the young girl is trading her body for dates, reassurance, or friends. Shame and guilt frequently occur.

If the young girl feels that sex is morally or religiously wrong, she may feel left out and lonely if all of her friends are having intercourse and she isn't. The double standard is another problem for girls. Boys in our culture are still encouraged to be more sexually active than girls.

With all these problems nurses are frequently placed in the position of adult confidant. This position can be used to good avail if we become educators and supportive models for teens. Nurses also need to be aware that different cultures place different values upon teenage pregnancy. In some cultures it is acceptable and part of the peer group values. In other cultures pregnancy is viewed as an act of rebellion or an attempt to separate from the parents.

Sadly, for some teens pregnancy is their only sense of belongingness and self-esteem: a child is their only possession. Studies have shown that when sex education programs focus on future opportunities and careers, or include parental involvement with teens, communication is improved and teenage pregnancy rates drop. School-based clinics, often run by nurses, have also been very successful in helping teenagers receive care.

Masturbation

Masturbation can safely be described as one of the most controversial sexual activities in Judaic-Christian culture. Masturbation is also the most common form of sexual outlet; some estimates are that as many as 94% of all men and 63% of all women masturbate. However, according to the Bible, Onan was killed for spilling his seed.

Many therapists, counselors, and health care professionals believe that masturbation is actually a healthy outlet for sexual expression, intimacy, and "getting to know one's body." However, many adolescents and adults experience a tremendous amount of anxiety, guilt, and shame when they masturbate.

It has also been theorized by Freud and other psychologists that masturbation triggers to a conscious level repressed (put away) fantasies from the Oedipal period—the period of time, identified by Freud, that occurs at approximately age 2 1/2. These feelings can be very traumatic and uncomfortable.

However, self-stimulation may serve sexuality in several beneficial ways. First, it may feel good. It also provides sexual release in a non-threatening way without the fear of pregnancy and sexually transmitted diseases. Finally, masturbation provides self-knowledge on what feels good—information that can eventually be shared with a partner.

Fantasy

Fantasizing is also another concern for the adolescent, but it can serve several positive purposes. It can be a pleasurable sexual activity and can also be used as a substitute for sexual intercourse or to enhance orgasm. Finally, fantasizing can serve as a means of sexual rehearsal and can also be a safe, unembarrassing way to disperse sexual energy.

Unfortunately, many adolescents and adults are taught that fantasizing, like masturbation, is immoral or abnormal. Teenagers typically have very little understanding of the meaning of fantasy. Therefore, if they experience a fantasy that is against their moral and cultural beliefs, they may feel shameful and guilty.

It is important to reaffirm that it is not necessarily true that when you have a fantasy you want that fantasy to be present in your everyday life. Fantasizing is a very helpful and pleasurable part of adult sexuality, and it is important that this experience is normalized.

Petting and Oral Sex

Petting, defined as "sexual touching below the waist," is also a very common activity for teenagers. Kinsey reported that by the age of 18, 80% of boys and girls had done some form of petting behavior.

Oral sex has also become much more common among teenagers. Recent studies show that as many as 50% of teenagers have engaged in oral sex. For many teenagers this sexual behavior seems "safer" than intercourse because there is no risk of pregnancy.

Illness-Related Sexual Problems

Adolescence is a difficult time to be acutely or chronically ill. Any acute episode of illness can trigger feelings of insecurity and cause regression. This can create a great amount of confusion for the adolescent who is coping with various stages of sexuality. Thus, the nurse must find the right balance of care, especially when sensitive body parts are involved. This can be a tricky juggling act at best and at worst may be traumatic for the nurse, the patient, and the family.

Any illness that results in a change in the physical appearance of the teenager is devastating. Frequently, it can hinder the expression of positive teenage sexuality because of the great desire to be similar to one's peer group.

Nonfatal diseases such as acne as well as catastrophic illnesses such as cancer can cause great anxiety. Learning to cope and adjust to the effects of treatment can be traumatic. These may include alopecia (the loss of hair), anorexia or weight gain, and mutilation caused by medications, chemotherapy, or surgical procedures and radiation. Scars and skin changes can be especially difficult experiences to cope with.

A little-acknowledged side-effect of chemotherapy, radiation, or surgery is infertility. At the onset of diagnosis, the staff, the parents, and the patient may be overwhelmed with decisions related to life and death, and decisions that affect the quality of life become delayed. But, infertility, which does affect the quality of life, can be a threat to self-esteem, body image, and also sexual concept. As nurses it is therefore important to keep in mind that the older adolescent may well be sexually mature and fertile. Options such as sperm banking and egg retrieval should be discussed. Sometimes it is difficult for professionals to get over their initial discomfort at addressing these issues. In some cases consulting a specialist in the fertility field can be helpful.

Hospitalized teenagers need to be given the permission to discuss all traumatic physical changes. Nurses can help by bringing in peers who have had the same experience. Having appropriate wigs and hairpieces available is also important. Finally, family and individual counseling related to these issues is crucial.

Implications for Nurses

It is very difficult for the adolescent to obtain health care for sexual concerns and problems. Since both parents and adolescents frequently are uncomfortable and feel embarrassed seeking out the expertise of health professionals, nurses can be important intermediaries because they are frequently trusted and respected by the patient and the physician.

Conversations about sexuality need to be tailored to the adolescents', social, emotional, and physical development. For medical and psychological reasons, it is also important to take a careful sex history. First, it is important to learn what the adolescent believes. Be aware of what values constitute his or her inner world. Adolescents typically get a clearer understanding of themselves through a discussion that helps clarify values and helps them make decisions.

Since many adolescents will not talk to an adult if they feel that the adult knows their parents or is a friend of their parents, it is important to reassure them about confidentiality. Confidentiality should always be respected unless the adolescent's safety or life is in jeopardy. Most parents are relieved to have a respected health professional involved with their child and will work cooperatively with you.

Adolescents also need nonjudgmental health teaching that includes accurate information about sexual health. Contraception, socially transmitted diseases, and AIDS, communication skills, and general health care are all topics that need to be discussed.

Adolescents need the opportunity to discuss issues related to sexual orientation. If they are gay, or are struggling with concerns about identity, they need a friendly, unbiased ear. Although sexologists still are debating the etiology of sexual orientation, frequently a brief discussion may greatly help allay the guilt a parent or adolescent may be feeling.

It is important not to label a teenager gay on the basis of an isolated sexual experience. Frequently teenagers just need timely information and the time and self-esteem to explore their sexuality in a nonjudgmental environment.

Adolescence can be a period of turmoil and fear, yet it can also be a time of tremendous growth and development. It is in many ways the springboard toward the maturation of intimacy and sexual expression. The nurse professional can help lead the way toward this maturity.

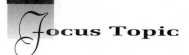

Focus Topic

What Teens Need to Know about Contraception and Sexually Transmitted Diseases (STDs) by Lori Cohen-Pasahow, BA, Ob/Gyn Family Planning CNP

The following discussion is based on almost 20 years of various work and volunteer experiences in women's health care. In my many individual and group experiences with teens I have found them to be open, creative, and entertaining when they are allowed to be just what they are: teens.

Throughout history women have taken steps to control their fertility. The earliest record of contraceptive use comes from 1850 B.C. Egyptian women used crocodile dung, food, honey pressed against the cervix, leaves pressed into a shape similar to the modern diaphragm, and lemon with the juice (lemon as a barrier and juice as a spermicide—Casanova's favorite).

Prior to the 1800s the major methods of contraception were vaginal sponges, tampons, douches (acidic juices, poisons), withdrawal, and abstinence. Self-induced abortion was another very dangerous option that was frequently used, as was infanticide.

Male methods of contraception included rubbing the penis with rock salt, tar, vinegar, onion juice, and other substances. Condoms made from a variety of different materials were also used. As early as 1350 B.C. Egyptians wore penile decorations which were forerunners of modern condoms.

Many methods of contraception were based on superstitions or folk beliefs. Here are some examples:

1. If a woman spits three times in a frog's mouth she will not conceive for a year.

2. Intercourse without passion does not lead to pregnancy.

3. Drinking teas made from fruitless trees will ensure "fruitlessness" (no pregnancy).

4. Coughing, sneezing, jumping up and down, or holding your nose and pushing hard forces semen out.

All of these "desperate and primitive acts," although some times quite ingenious, speak to the fact that women have always wanted fertility control. Yet not until the late 19th century did contraception and family planning develop. Finally, in 1873, condoms and diaphragms were available to women seeing a physician for a prescription. Early condoms were first constructed from animal intestines and were popularized by none other than Casanova.

Our values and attitudes are the framework through which we see the world. The mix of race, religion, education, economic standing, family size and dynamics, geographics, and community forms certain attitudes, beliefs, and values, including those related to sexuality. Family planning decisions and behaviors result from the development of these values. Therefore, it's important for nurses to recognize and accept values that are different from theirs. Our duty is to simply help our patients clarify their values and consider the behavioral options that are open to them.

For instance, if a 14-year-old comes in telling you that she thinks she has an infection because she has pain and a foul discharge, and she is having unprotected sex, it is important to recognize what this 14-year-old is asking of you and not just dictate what you think she really needs. If you have strong religious feelings which prevent you from recommending certain methods, you need to be aware of this limitation. Perhaps you are uncomfortable working in this area, or perhaps your feelings, beliefs, and background limit your ability to give all of the needed information in an unbiased fashion. Be sure to listen to yourself, because the messages given by professionals should be value free.

In all these situations, just give the facts accurately and listen; do not impose judgment on the teen's behavior or requests. When you give value judgments, the teen turns you off and doesn't come back. Remember, it takes a lot of courage for a young woman or man to come to your agency, hospital, or emergency room, to receive treatment for a sexually transmitted disease or to seek birth control. These clients count on us for accurate information and treatment in a confidential, nonjudgmental manner.

Adolescence is a time of stress, both physiologically and psychologically. It is a time for changing, growing, trying out new behaviors, and discovering a place in the world. Emotions are volatile, and the sense of self is in flux. Peer groups often take the place of families, and bodies begin to look and feel different.

Faced with this turmoil, professionals need to look at themselves closely and examine their reactions, motivations, and biases. Ultimately, they are the ones who become the advocates for the teen, and this relationship must be built on trust if the teen is to come back. Confidentiality is therefore very important. When we lose a teen, we risk increasing all of those problems that face them, such as unintended pregnancies and sexually transmitted diseases, which can lead to infertility. We also lose the connection to help them in future situations.

The most common and popular goals of sexually active teens include preventing unintended pregnancy and treating and preventing sexually transmitted diseases. However, they may not be presented this way, because teenagers generally perceive these concerns as entangled with other problems, such as acne, depression, anxiety, eating disorders, sexual questions, parents, friends, alcohol, drugs, and school. These differences in perception can be frustrating for nurses who struggle with compliance and responsibility issues, and also for teenagers who may feel that their most pressing needs are not being adequately addressed. For example, the nurse who carefully describes risks, benefits, and side-effects may find that for the teen the greatest perceived risk is "getting caught" and being embarrassed.

Another point to remember is that patients come to see health care providers with knowledge and attitudes formed from the media, personal experiences, family, and peers. They may be well versed in contraceptive knowledge or dangerously misinformed. In any case, it is a mistake to assume, that they get most of their health information from a doctor's office or clinic. When you have adolescents as patients you may have a very short time to actually find out what they know and then help them unlearn all of the misinformation as well as learn what they genuinely want and need to know.

The mass media definitely influence attitudes toward contraception. The kinds of messages teens receive are sometimes the principles by which they learn about contraception, and they may form incorrect attitudes. One survey has shown that in the course of a year the average viewer sees more than 9,000 scenes of sexual intercourse or innuendo on prime-time TV. Our young people are barraged by the message "sophistication equals being sexually hip." We don't even buy toothpaste because it is an effective method of fighting tooth decay; we buy it to be sexually attractive.

Thus the teen hears many messages from friends and advertisements. Here is a sampling of the myths that result from these messages:

1. An advertisement says that this product "contains no hormones," and therefore it is better. This translates to "hormones are bad for you—don't use them.

2. A woman's body needs a "rest" from birth control pills. Many women come in asking this question: "Don't I need to take a rest?" And I say, "When you take a rest, you get a pregnancy-induced rest!"

3. "Won't I get breast cancer if I use birth control pills?" The media stress bad news and focus on the punitive.

4. "I can't get pregnant when I have my period or have breakthrough bleeding."

5. "I can't get pregnant the first time that I have sex or if I have it occasionally, or standing up."

6. A woman should douche after her period because she's not "clean" at that time and women are supposed to smell like flowers.

A strategy for addressing these issues are to counsel patients carefully, lists risks and benefits, listen to their questions, and answer them honestly to allay their fears. Listening means paying attention to every cue: listening with your eyes as well as your ears. This is a way to show that you care. How many times do we hear teens say, "No one listens"?

Most teens deny that they are sexually active. Moreover, sexual involvement is not clearly connected with pregnancy. Attitudes include, "I didn't know it could happen to me," "It won't happen to me," and "If it happens it happens." Or you may have the teen who says, "It [sex] only happened twice and my mom thinks it's happening every day." Young people find it difficult to admit to themselves that they are having sexual intercourse. They prefer to think it is something that just happens. They need to understand that the first step in assuming responsibility for their sexual behavior is to recognize that becoming or not becoming sexually involved is a choice (their choice).

Often sexual intercourse is a means of achieving something else. Teenage girls are likely to say, "I had sex because my boyfriend would find someone else if I didn't." Boys and girls may say, "I thought all of my friends were having sex, and I wanted to be part of the crowd," or, "I was afraid if I didn't have sex I wouldn't be popular" or "I wouldn't feel grown up."

In the eyes of their peers, it is important for teens to be sexually active. That may be a hard thing for you, the nurse, to accept. "No one wants to be a virgin": there can be a lot of pressure even on a 14-year-old. Again, the media help perpetuate this attitude. Yet adolescents wait approximately 1 year between the time they being having sexual intercourse and the time they begin using contraceptives. One-third of the women who seek birth control are teens. In 1985 the single most common reason for girls between the ages of 15 and 20 to visit a physician was for prenatal care. Therefore, nurses need to use every opportunity to teach identity formation, personal and family values identification, sex roles, goal setting, decision making, and communication skills. All of this will help develop understanding and prepare the teen for parenthood, adult sexuality, and personal growth.

The most common questions posed by teens include the following:

How can I get birth control without my parents' knowledge?

How can I say no?

How can I enjoy sex more?

How can I tell that I am pregnant?

How can I avoid pregnancy?

Can a guy tell if I have had sex before?

Don't I need a "cleaning" or "dusting" once in a while? (Patients are really asking if they need a routine dilatation and curettage.)

How can I tell if he had his "wick" where it don't belong?

How do I know if a guy has had the "drip" before?

Aren't I supposed to douche every time after I have sex?

Am I supposed to have a discharge?

Is sex supposed to feel good, or it supposed to hurt?

Choosing the right method of answering these question can be difficult. We all have our rap: contraceptive alternative rap, pregnancy decision rap, sexually transmitted diseases, AIDS, drugs. We often feel frustrated when we see that our teens are not learning the information that we present. Sometimes they do understand the information but they do not use it to influence their choices. It is important to remember that we are not responsible for their *decisions*; however, as professionals we need to know that we have done the best that we can.

The following is part of an interview demonstrating a nurse trying to understand a teen better:

Nurse: "Can you tell me what's confusing you?"

Teen: "There's no method for me."

Nurse: "What do you mean there's no method for you?"

Teen: "I just know that none will work for me."

At this point you could run through your usual information speech, or...

Nurse: "Can you describe what you know about each method and what the problem is?"

Contraceptive Methods

Listed below are contraceptive methods with a brief description of each. Remember, the most common question is, "Will it work?"

Norplant: This is available as a long-acting (5 years) contraceptive which consists of six Silastic capsules inserted in a fanlike pattern under the dermis on the upper inside portion of the arm. It is presently the most effective birth control option because its effectiveness is 99.5%.

Oral contraceptives: This is the most popular method and has been used for more than 30 years. Oral contraceptives, or birth control pills (BCPs), contain the synthetic hormones estrogen and progesterone and are effective in preventing ovulation. There are over 12 million pill users worldwide. Some of the commonly asked questions regarding BCPs include the following:

My partner doesn't want me to take BCPs. What should I do?

Can I drink alcohol or take drugs with BCPs?

I'm on a low-dose BCP, so am I protected enough?

How long can I take the BCP?

IUD (intrauterine device): This is a small device inserted by a doctor or nurse practitioner into the uterus. There are several types available. They include the Copper Seven, the Copper-T, and the Safety-coil. Currently only 2% of the women in the United States use the IUD, although 84 million worldwide use it. Some common questions include the following:

Can my partner feel the string?

How do I know that everything is okay and that the IUD is in?

What happens if I get pregnant with the IUD?

How often should I replace the IUD?

Diaphragm and cervical cap: The diaphragm is a dome-shaped, shallow rubber cup with a flexible rim. The cervical cap is a small, thimble-shaped latex cup. Before inserting, use spermicidal jelly or cream around the rim and inside to increase effectiveness. The diaphragm acts as a plate up against the cervix. It is one of the few methods over which a woman has complete control, since she can remove and insert it at will. It should be fitted by a physician or nurse practitioner.

Sponge: This is another barrier method which is also nonprescriptive. It is permeated with spermacidal nonoxynol-9. Thus it blocks the cervix and is also effective against sexually transmitted diseases.

Contraceptive foams, creams, jellies, suppositories: all of these contain nonoxynol-9. This method decreases sexually transmitted diseases and protects against pelvic inflammatory disease (PID). No doctor's visit or prescription is needed. One disadvantage that is important to discuss with teens is that some may have a bad taste with oral sex. However, the jellies are tasteless.

Condoms: These are available in a variety of colors, shapes, and styles. All prevent pregnancy and in most cases sexually transmitted diseases, with the exception of AIDS. It is very important to educate teens how to use a condom. A helpful tip for an adolescent boy who is resistant about the condom is to remind him that condoms may slow down ejaculation because of decreased sensation. For the adolescent boy who "comes" too fast this may be very helpful. Condoms are very inexpensive, very accessible, and effective when used with cream or jelly.

Abstinence: This is 100% safe, has no costs, or side-effects, and eliminates risks, sexually transmitted diseases, worries, and conflict with parents.

Sterilization: This is permanent contraception. Tubal ligation and vasectomy are the most common methods of sterilization. They are 99% effective and should be considered irreversible. They do not affect sexual pleasure or sensation in any way. Some common questions include the following:

Is sterilization reversible?

What happens to the egg or sperm?

Will sterilization affect femininity or masculinity?

Will anyone be able to tell that I have had sterilization without my telling them?

Will I have less of a sex drive?

Does sterilization cause cancer?

Will it make my periods heavier?

In conclusion, our responsibility is to give the message that sex has consequences and that some of these consequences can be harmful (see Table 4–1). However, we should not let our message become "sex is bad."

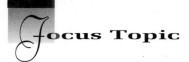

Focus Topic

Chronic Disease and the Adolescent

Children with chronic conditions may differ from healthy children in terms of physical growth. However, in terms of sexuality their needs to explore and express themselves are comparable to those of healthy children. Health care professionals who work with chronically ill adolescents frequently fail to address issues regarding sexual development and sexual responsibility.

Helping children and families live as normal a life as possible is an important goal. This may be very difficult for the child who is isolated or separated from peers. Information regarding sex and sexuality therefore needs to be included in the care plan for the child.

Unfortunately, sexuality is often only equated with healthy children, not the disabled, and material written for the disabled child is almost nonexistent. This is a tragedy, because it is foolish to assume that children with chronic diseases do not try to seek out sexual experiences.

Chronic illness, on top of the normal developmental challenges, can make the physically and mentally disabled child ignorant of useful information and prone to risk-taking behavior. Pregnancy, child abuse, abortion, prostitution, and sexually transmitted diseases can result. Unfortunately, disabled children who have poor self-esteem caused by their negative physical self-image are especially vulnerable to the negative consequences of sexually inappropriate behavior.

Table 4–1
Socially & Sexually Transmitted Diseases

Signs & Symptoms	Possible Causes	Transmission of Disease	Signs Usually Show Up By	Possible Consequences
Burning and/or discharge (drip) from sex organs	Gonorrhea (clap, drip, dose)	Sexual contact with infected person.	1–30 days	Arthritis, blindness, sterility. Prostate problems in men. Pelvic inflammatory disease in women.
	Non-Gonococcal Urethritis		1–3 weeks	Babies can be infected at birth and develop pneumonia and blindness.
	Trichomonas (Trich)	Sexual contact with infected person or use of contaminated articles such as towels and washcloths.	4–28 days	Gland infection or damage to women's sex organs. Painful intercourse. Unknown in men.
	Monilia (Yeast)	Overgrowth of yeast fungus normally present in women's vaginas. Men get it by having sex with infected women.	Varies	Can be passed to newborn causing severe infection. Painful intercourse.
	Gardnerella Vaginitis	Sexual contact with infected person or use of contaminated articles.	Varies	Rarely leads to any serious complications.
Severe lower stomach pain, nausea, fever	Pelvic Inflammatory Disease	(In women only) Sexual contact with male infected with Gonorrhea or Non-Gonococcal Urethritis.	2 weeks–2 months	Sterility, long term stomach pain, tubal damage, tubal pregnancy.
Severe itching and bumps on and around sex organs	Scabies	Sexual contact with infected person or use of contaminated articles such as towels, bed, comb.	1–2 weeks	Other infections caused by the intense scratching of infected area.
	Lice (Crabs)		1–6 weeks	
	Trich and Yeast		Varies	
Painful sores or blisters on sex organs	Herpes	Sexual contact with infected person.	Varies	Can be passed to newborn and cause severe illness and death.
	Chancroid		2–6 days	Other germs can infect open sores and cause additional infection.
Painless sores on sex organs or rashes	Syphilis	Sexual contact with infected person. Pregnant woman can pass it to unborn child.	10–90 days	Blindness, insanity, nerve problems, heart disease, stillbirth, death.
Nausea, vomiting, diarrhea, bloody stools	Giardiasis	Oral-rectal sexual contact (rimming) with infected person.	Few days–Few months	Recurring stomach cramps, prolonged diarrhea, dehydration.
	Amebiasis			
	Shigellosis		1–7 days	
Growths on sex organs	Venereal Warts	Sexual contact with infected person.	1–3 months	Large growths can cause blockage of rectal and vaginal openings.
Yellow skin and eyes, dark urine	Hepatitis B	Sexual or other intimate contact with infected person.	1–4 months	Liver problems.

Source: The New Jersey State Department of Health Sexually Transmitted Disease Control.

Health Care Assessment

The health care assessment is an important tool for understanding the needs of these adolescents. Muscari (1987) provides the following guidelines for taking a successful sexual history of the adolescent:

1. Be accepting and nonjudgmental of the adolescent's sexual attitudes and preferences.

2. Provide privacy.

3. Demonstrate a caring attitude.

4. Maintain eye contact.

5. Identify the motives behind the adolescent's sexual activity.

6. Promote trust by providing confidentiality.

7. Assess both the adolescent's sexual development and his or her sexual practices.

Problems Related to Sexual Expression

There are many different problems related to the expression of sexuality for adolescents with chronic disease.

Pain: For example, children with juvenile rheumatoid arthritis (JRA) may have temporomandibular joint pain with kissing. Because of the joint stiffness that accompanies JRA, they may also have difficulty with touching and even positioning themselves to insert birth control devices.

The teenage male with sickle-cell anemia may experience the pain related to priapism, or curvature of the penis during an erection. Teenagers who have leukemia may have joint, gland, and bone pain.

Motor instability: Children with cerebral palsy may experience altered balance and posturing, as well as difficulty with relaxing. Drooling is another problem, and may interfere with the child's ability to experiment sexually as well as with the partner's desire for intimacy. The inability to control movements or speech can influence social interaction, and the child with spinal cord injury may not be able to move at all.

Offensive odors: The presence of "offensive" odors can hinder intimacy and create a negative sense of self. Situations that may cause this problem include cystic fibrosis, colostomies or ureterostomies, and altered bowel and bladder function.

Altered body image: There are many different situations that may help create a negative perception of body image. Illnesses, congenital defects, and treatment of illness can all create body image changes. Surgical alterations such as colostomy or amputations cause obvious changes that will trigger anxiety. In rheumatoid arthritis the child may develop swollen joints that are unsightly, and the child with systemic lupus erythematosus may develop ugly rashes, hair loss, and swollen joints.

Other conditions may cause an alteration in taste and temperature, paralysis, or decreased ability to have an erection. Some conditions may cause changes in libido or a change in body shape. Teenagers who are on cortisone may become very heavy and sometimes depressed. Alopecia (hair loss), whether natural or the result of treatment, can be devastating for the teenager.

As a result of these problems, teenagers may develop psychological problems related to self-esteem, isolation or withdrawal, rebellion, and even shame.

Nursing Interventions

Interventions are based upon an assessment that takes into account at least some of the following issues: the patients' prior coping skills, their support system, and their sense of self-esteem. Other issues include their goals and dreams for the future, the prognosis of the disease, and their culture. Interventions need to be customized to fit the needs of the patient. General rules for beginning to approach this subject include the following (Selekman, 1991):

1. Be sensitive to the cultural beliefs and practices of the child.

2. Have a nonjudgmental attitude regarding the child's lack of sexual knowledge.

3. Anticipate questions.

4. Differentiate between normal adolescent behaviors and how the child is behaving.

5. Allow the adolescent to take an active part in any planning of his or her sexual health.

Specific suggestions include the following:

1. Share accurate information. This may include specific suggestions to enhance sexual activity, such as showering and bathing, emptying the bladder, and using moist heat for the pain of arthritis.

2. Help the adolescent feel comfortable asking questions.

3. Arrange for peer counseling by a slightly older person of the same sex. One of the issues of children with chronic disease is that they may have fewer social opportunities than others and cannot go to the usual places where teenagers typically socialize and hang out.

4. Help create a positive body image by teaching the adolescent how to dress appropriately in appealing clothes and jewelry, how to use makeup, and how to follow good grooming tips.

5. Teach teenagers to meet the needs of their significant others in ways other than through sexual intercourse. Stress that there are other ways to foster loving and caring relationships.

A closing note on parents of children with chronic diseases: Many parents are very uncomfortable talking to their children about sexuality. Yet they need to share their values and cultural beliefs with their children. It is a difficult balancing act to be both the advocate for the child and to not have the parents feel as if we are overstepping our boundary and taking their role. Many parents actually need the same kind of information as their children.

Hopefully, we can be advocates for adolescents with a chronic disease and therefore give them the opportunity to express themselves in a positive and age-appropriate manner.

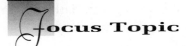

Focus Topic

An Overview of Adolescence

Object-relations theory: Idealized peer and idol attachments. Teens try on new roles and identities. This is sometimes called the second separation as adolescents struggle to separate from their parents and their parents struggle with allowing them to separate.

Freud/late genital period: Beginning of genitally focused sexuality.

Erikson/identity versus identity confusion: Basic modality is to lose self and find self in another. Transition from childhood to adulthood is not typically smooth. Adolescent questions ideals and beliefs of parental figures. Needs to separate from parents and create satisfactory relations with opposite sex. Begins to decide on a vocation. Relationships are increasingly important.

Stage in family life cycle: Some children may be beginning to leave home.

Sexuality: Creation of satisfactory relations and intimacy with opposite sex. Acceptance of new body image after rapid growth. Beginning of puberty: first menses, growth of breasts, first ejaculation, growth of pubic hair. Attitudes toward masturbation important. Voice changes and beards develop for boys. Both males and females experience a maximum growth spurt. Clearer concept of sexual orientation: which gender they are attracted to.

Stressors related to illness: Body image challenges due to illness, embarrassment, modesty, isolation from peer group, threats to sexuality, fear of infertility, increased dependence on parents, separation from school, regression, anger.

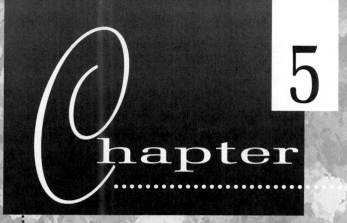

Chapter 5

Early Adulthood:
An Adventure
in Intimacy

Mary Ellen sat and stared out of the window. It was a cold brisk day. She closed her eyes and began to think about last night. It had been perfect. They had spent hours talking and dancing. Finally, they had begun to make love. Yes, it had been perfect until the baby starting screaming. Jack had been upset. He couldn't understand why she just didn't ignore the baby's crying; he could. Jack had finally just turned on his back and gone to sleep. What could Mary Ellen do? Did she have to chose? Who could she talk to?

Early adulthood ushers in both privileges and responsibilities. The young adult needs to make many important decisions regarding relationships, careers, and life-style. Early adulthood is not only a "critical" time for experiencing new relationships but for some individuals a time for making a commitment to one person for what is considered to be the rest of their lives.

No longer children in the developmental sense of the word, young adults move out of their parents' homes to live with newfound lovers or spouses. Many young women need to decide whether to start a family, stay in school, or develop a career. For young adults who are not heterosexual, early adulthood is the period when they begin to feel more comfortable with their sexual orientation.

Although young adults can be confronted with a catastrophic illness such as cancer, diabetes, or AIDS, the majority do not get sick. Typically the nurse's contact with them is for contraceptive advice, prenatal care, or an acute illness or accident. Counseling issues are frequently related to relationships and intimacy.

PSYCHOSOCIAL TASKS

According to Erikson, early adulthood is the critical time period for determining whether a person will be successful in developing a capacity for intimacy and caring for others. He termed this sixth stage of his theory *intimacy versus isolation*. Erikson believed that if young adults are not successful in this developmental task, they may well remain isolated from the "dance of intimacy."

The normal march of time typically reinforces and augments for the young adult the biological, psychological, and sociological influences of adolescence. Frequently, however, some emotional issues and concerns of childhood and adolescence still need to be integrated and understood. Many young adults struggle to consolidate and validate their earlier emotional experiences.

Developing a more mature sense of self may mean adjusting to new cultural sex roles versus the older, more traditional behaviors that until recently were expected of young adults. Although these traditional expectations are now changing, it is the author's observation that many men and women still believe and practice traditional sex role behavior: that is, during these adult years men continue to be more career focused and women are still more relationship and family focused.

Some women are still raised to feel that their futures are linked to the occupational success of their husbands. A growing number of women, however, are choosing a different developmental route and are seeking careers that form an inherent part of their identity. Many women are now becoming professionals and are entering nursing, law, business administration, engineering, and medicine. Unfortunately, American culture has still not developed the societal supports to enable these women to manage dual lives as both career women and mothers. As a consequence, finding time to pursue their own health care may be stressful for women who are juggling work, marriage, and children. Finally, nurses need to be sensitive to the negative attitudes our culture has for women who solely parent. Many of these women feel that society does not consider them "worthy" as "working women."

SEXUAL EXPRESSION

The sexual expression of the young adult usually does not differ significantly from that of the sexually active adolescent. However, sexual activity does increase. Young adulthood is also a period of sexual experimentation.

Many adults now live away from their parents and so have more privacy and less restraint. Possibly as a result of this distance, there seems to be a greater degree of comfort with premarital sexuality. This independence may encourage more differentiation and separation from the parents. Young adults are no longer extensions of their family of origin but are living on their own.

Accessible contraception now makes possible sex for pleasure without procreation and therefore lowers the fear of becoming pregnant. Sexual activity for pleasure rather than just for procreation is at least superficially approved by our culture, and this attitude encourages more sexual expression outside marriage. Whether or not nurses approve, nurse professionals should be nonjudgmental when discussing sexual expression with young adults.

Although many young adults are comfortable in seeking the stability of a primary intimate relationship, others are not as developmentally mature in their sexuality and intimacy skills. Those who are insecure may avoid intimacy.

There are many reasons why there may be sexual performance anxiety for the young adult. One reason is that sex is frequently used as a proving ground for masculinity or femininity. For some men, sex elicits fear of inadequate performance. Other men fear that they are incapable of satisfying a woman. Young women may also share these concerns. Some are fearful that they cannot "attract" and "hold" a male.

Homophobic behaviors can also be experienced. Fears regarding homosexuality or fear of being a homosexual may cause concern. Other anxiety-producing issues include equating sexual virility or feminine attraction with the number of men or women with whom one has had sex. Concerns regarding frequency can also contribute to sexual compulsive behavior, conflict, and performance anxiety.

Contemporary women may also have to cope with performance anxiety regarding orgasm. Some may be fearful of being anorgasmic. The media contribute to this anxiety by sending constant messages regarding sexual expectations and expression. Whether the orgasm is vaginal or clitoral may also cause a great amount of concern. Unfortunately, many men and women still believe Freud's theory that clitoral orgasms are "immature." However, present research indicates that the clitoris is the most potent erotic part of the genitalia for women and is typically where orgasm originates.

Men frequently have fears related to impotency or premature ejaculation. Our culture perpetuates the myth that men must always be ready to perform sexually. Men, according to some of the popular literature, must be sexually "like a machine" and must also be multiorgasmic.

Nurses need to understand that myths regarding ideal male and female sexuality abound and frequently color the self-perceptions of adults. Many men and women are affected by these erroneous myths and unfortunately judge their sexuality by standards that are rigid, unrealistic, and ultimately traumatic.

SEXUALITY AND MARRIAGE

Traditionally, marriage has been a stabilizing factor in our culture. Because most adults (90%) choose to be married at some time during their life cycle, it is important for the nurse to be aware of some of the concerns that marriage can create. These include true love versus being taken for granted, fidelity versus lack of commitment, pleasuring the partner and self versus sexual dysfunction, and time for children versus time for their lover. Sexual dysfunctions such as anorgasmia, premature ejaculation, erectile dysfunction, and lack of desire may be present at various times during the life cycle.

Destructive intergenerational communication styles, intolerant in-laws, mixed religious marriages, differences in the need for and variety of sexual activity, and conflicts in moral and ethical decision making may also be experienced. Cultural variations in terms of sexual expression, changing sex roles, different communication styles, and ignorance of sexual techniques are other common concerns and areas of conflict.

All of these concerns are further influenced by work, excess or more frequently lack of money, and parental, peer, and parenting stress. Infidelity and divorce are frequent results of these problems. Some of the latest studies seem to indicate that couples married under 4 years are at very high risk for divorcing.

Another important obstacle influencing marital stability is the lack of accurate and timely information for young couples who are marrying. American culture does not provide many services or much education related to premarital counseling, communication skills, or even values clarification for couples. As a result of this dearth of material, many couples enter marriage with little understanding of their own emotional issues and expectations regarding their spouse and marriage in general.

Although most nurses are not trained in marriage and family therapy skills, they need to be aware of those experts in their geographic area who can be of help to their patients. For example, a marriage and family therapist could be a psychiatrist, a psychologist, or a clinical nurse specialist such as the author. By taking a careful psychosocial history, we can better identify those men and women who are at higher risk for divorce. Premarital or marital therapy may be very helpful to these couples.

Sexual problems may also occur as the novelty of marriage wears off or as the emotional adjustment necessary for living with another person becomes too difficult. As a result of these adaptations, sex may become less gratifying and exciting. In fact, recent research is indicating that the frequency of sexual intercourse may go from as much as 14.8 times per month in the newly married couple to only 6.6 times by the 6th year of marriage. Therapists are still debating whether sexual problems occur as the result of a troubled relationship or vice versa.

There are many causes of sexual dysfunction in the young adult. These may include anxiety, fear of failure, excessive need to please the partner, unrealistic expectations, great personal demands, discomfort in abandoning oneself to erotic pleasure out of fear of performance, poor self-esteem, prior sexual abuse and/or incest, physical pain, poor communication skills, religious and cultural messages, lack of relationship skills. Any one of these issues may affect a marriage in a negative way.

PREGNANCY

The announcement of a pregnancy is hopefully the result of a healthy progression from the establishment of an intimate relationship to the creation of a new generation. However, pregnancy requires enormous adjustments for the individual and the spouse in terms of sexual expression, sex role expectations, and other intrapsychic challenges.

The arrival of the first child often forces young parents to take that last major step into the adult world. They now are totally responsible for the emotional and physical needs of another person.

For all generations within the family, the birth of a child affects and changes relationships. Parenthood changes the family from a dyad to a unit of at least three individuals. It is a major transitional phase in the development of the couple, and therefore necessitates a great amount of adjustment and work. Unfortunately, our culture perpetuates a myth that pregnancy and childbirth are "romantic," and does not address some of the major issues that are helpful for couples to understand and cope with when a pregnancy occurs.

Sexuality During Pregnancy

This section examines some of the issues related to sexuality throughout the maternity cycle.

Despite the obvious importance of sexual activity during pregnancy, there is very little available data on how people cope with their sexuality during pregnancy. Perhaps this lack of research reflects our cultural uneasiness with the idea of sexuality and motherhood in the same person. For some people *lover* and *mother* feel like two very incongruous terms. Actually, human beings are the only mammals that have sexual activity during pregnancy. All other mammals refrain from sex during this time.

Because children are an important part of our culture, we like to perpetuate and romanticize the notion that pregnancy is typically a joyful period of time for a couple. The reality is that often it is not. This may be due to numerous factors, including unresolved marital issues, family of origin issues, economic concerns, and intrapsychic feelings regarding becoming a parent.

It takes time and experience to be able to interpret some of the many different kinds of feelings and emotions that couples experience during pregnancy. However, it is undisputed that pregnancy changes the very dynamics of a couple's relationship in both positive and negative ways. For some women, for example, pregnancy, elicits strong feelings of dependency and may be an especially confusing time for the woman who has valued her sense of independence. Some men react with anger and resentment to the behaviors that result. If the couple does not share with the nurse that there are some relationship problems occurring in the marriage and the nurse does not pick up the nonverbal messages that the couple is bringing to the health care setting, these problems may not be discussed. The sexual well-being of the couple should be of concern to their medical caregivers. Pregnancy is an invaluable opportunity for assessing and teaching the couple about physical and emotional changes that will occur.

The first detailed study of sexual activity during pregnancy was part of the work of William M. Masters and Virginia Johnson (1966). Masters and Johnson studied 101 multiparas and primiparas. They reported an initial decrease in coital desire and frequency in the first trimester of pregnancy. In the second trimester, they found that there was some increase in sexual interest and performance as the pelvic vasculature experienced more congestion. However, by the third trimester, Masters and Johnson reported a major drop in both sexual interest and activity. This lack of desire and activity continued for 50% of the respondents for at least 3 months after delivery. It is impossible to determine how much of the reported lack of desire was due to fatigue and the psychological tensions of caring for a child. Other studies have also found similar behavior patterns.

Masters and Johnson also questioned women regarding their beliefs as to why their sexual experiences changed during pregnancy. The reasons that they gave included, physical discomfort (46%), fear of injury to the baby (27%), loss of interest (23%), physician suggestion (8%), and sense of loss of attractiveness (1%).

Although the conflict regarding whether it was okay to be sexual and pregnant did not come up in these respondents' answers, I suggest that on some level this concern may have caused a conflict. What is important for us to realize for both our patients and their significant others is that frequently they may not be aware of the normalcy of this lack of desire. As a result, the spouse, who is himself undergoing many stresses caused by the pregnancy, may react to his wife's withdrawal with loss and pain. Therefore, the nurse should be sure that couples are aware of the probability of this lack of desire. Without this knowledge the male may internalize this experience as rejection or abandonment.

Another interesting phenomenon that occurs occasionally is that expectant fathers complain that they have many of the same symptoms of pregnancy that their wife is having. This intense over-identification may cause these men to experience backache, nausea, and weight gain.

For most couples it is also good to give practical tips and suggestions for coping with the changing body of the pregnant women and still remaining sexual. Unfortunately, many couples are embarrassed to ask the kinds of questions that could be helpful to them. Therefore, as nurses we need to help create an environment which can make them feel at ease and give them the courage to ask about sexual concerns. Probably the most consistent change in sexual behavior for the couple is coital position. Most couples change from the missionary position (man on top of woman) to either a side-by-side or rear-entry position. As intercourse becomes more difficult, there are other options available for the couple that are safe and satisfying. These include masturbation and oral sex.

Potential Dangers

Although this has been a great concern for many, studies have not shown a relationship between coital activity and premature labor. However, certain medical conditions do have a potential for causing premature labor. These include mechanical failures such as an opened cervix, infections, and uterine excessive contractions.

Many couples are fearful that the thrusting of the penis in the vagina can cause ruptured membranes, or placental bleeding. Although this fear is widespread, no research has affirmed its validity. It is felt that the baby, surrounded by the amniotic fluid, is very safe from penile thrusting.

However, vaginal bleeding is an important reason not to have intercourse. Other reasons to abstain include a healing vaginal or surgical wound that just happens to coincide with pregnancy. Infection is another contraindication. A woman who has an incompetent cervical os (a cervix that is not fully closed), ruptured membranes, or a dilated cervix late in pregnancy could develop an infection from sexual intercourse. These women need to refrain from sexual intercourse.

Another concern of some couples is related to fear of orgasm. Because orgasm produces uterine contractions, women who have had premature births or have a dilated cervix, and who have orgasm during sex, may be at greater risk for going into premature labor. It is judicious to educate these couples about the inherent risks of orgasm. Actually, any woman late in her pregnancy can bring on labor when she has an orgasm. Non-orgasmic sexual behavior, however, is usually safe.

Cunnilingus may be a dangerous sexual activity if the partner forces air in the vagina. This "blowing air" to "cool" the vagina causes an air embolism which can cause death as it travels up the veins, through the heart, and then lodges in the lungs.

Although this list is actually quite small, it is important for nurses to educate patients as to when sex could be dangerous. Unfortunately, historically this danger has been exaggerated and misunderstood.

POSTPARTUM PERIOD

Sexuality

Noncoital sex can be resumed almost immediately after birth. However, women's interest in sex during the post-partum period is usually very low. Some couples may even feel awkward after the birth of the baby and may need some form of permission to resume sexual activities. Fatigue often contributes to this sexual disinterest.

As a result of some of the interpsychic conflicts discussed earlier, sexuality does not always return to prepregnancy levels. For many couples, therefore, sex after pregnancy is a major readjustment. Physical changes influences this adjustment as well as the emotional turmoil that the experience of birth signifies.

A common physiological problem related to the postpartum period is vaginal dryness caused by estrogen deprivation in the vagina. This is a normal hyposecretory response. It is completely independent of the female's psychological level of sexual responsiveness and is purely a physiological response. Patients and their partners may need to be educated about this phenomenon. Estrogen depletion is usually self-limiting and adjusts by the third postpartum month. However, it can cause some couples relationship problems; especially if it is misinterpreted as reflecting lack of sexual or partner interest. Patients may need to be told about the use of additional lubricants such as water-soluble creams. For the non-nursing mother estrogen creams can be very helpful. However, nursing mothers should not use estrogen cream because it can be absorbed into the blood stream and be expressed through the mother's milk.

Nursing mothers may also have concerns regarding their sexual functioning. They may feel uncomfortable with their body because they frequently retain extra fat. If their partner values slenderness, this may also be a problem for him. Body image changes may be difficult to adjust to, and frequently a negative body image will lower sexual desire and interest.

Persisting low levels of estrogen may also make the genitals extremely sensitive. In addition, the breasts may be sore and tender from nursing. Fatigue may be very high since nursing babies are fed through the night. Any of these physiological processes can inhibit intimacy.

Psychosocial Implications of Becoming a Parent

The birth a baby can be a mixed blessing for the sexual health of a couple. Childbirth and child care can place severe stresses on the new mother. She may feel fatigued or overwhelmed with the new responsibility. The new baby may also be a complete distraction for her, and her bonding with the child may make her partner feel excluded. Old behaviors and feelings originating from her own and the father's family of origin may once again come to the surface when they become parents. Even choosing the baby's name can cause major family battles.

The partner may feel excluded and overwhelmed. The birth of a baby may bring back both good and bad memories for him. Some men have a very difficult time adjusting from being part of a couple to becoming part of a family. Financial stresses may also become more severe, and for many partners the birth of a baby necessitates finding more work.

Grandparenting issues also may intrude upon the boundaries of this newly formed family. Frequent visits from proud grandparents can be helpful but may also lessen the period of time the couple has to be alone. Frequently, time becomes very pressured, and the couple has little time or energy to renegotiate and reconciliate. This can be very destructive for not only intimate communication but also for sexuality.

LOSS OF A CHILD

As many as 40% of pregnancies end in abortion or miscarriage. If the couple is not given permission to grieve the loss of the child, this experience can cause havoc with not only their relationship but also their sexual life.

Women who have delivered stillborn infants have suffered the death of a child. Sex may then become symbolically poignant to them and remind them of their loss. They may also be fearful of becoming pregnant again and may avoid sex for that reason. Anger and depression can also contribute to loss of desire and may be experienced by both the mother and father. If there are other siblings in the home, they too will need to grieve. It is very important to include the children in the grieving process; although children grieve differently than adults, allowing them to work through this loss is crucial for their mental well-being.

Such a loss may also contribute to a sense of body image distortion. The body does not know that the child died; therefore, the mother's milk may come in. Also, all of the dramatic physical changes regarding postpartum physiology may also occur, including a normal lack of desire. All of these variables can contribute to sexual and marital dysfunction. Nurses need to be aware of these implications and be available for educating, and counseling. They can also refer the couple to resource groups such as Resolve Through Sharing, a national support group for women and men who have lost a child.

In conclusion, pregnancy and the postpartum period herald in a new time and movement toward increased opportunities to be a family. However, these changes are monumental and require enormous physical and psychological coping skills. As nurse professionals we are in a very important position to help our clients negotiate this time in a healthy and successful manner. Reproduction is one of human beings' overriding concerns.

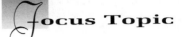

Focus Topic

What Happened to the American Family?

The American family is changing rapidly. Therefore, the support systems and the responsibilities of our patients are also changing. No longer can health professionals make any assumptions about the composition of any patient's family. For example, let's examine the following statistics.

1. Married couples with children dropped from 44% of American households to 27% between 1960 and 1988.

2. The average number of children per couple is 1.8.

3. Single-parent households from 1960 to 1988 increased by 13%. This is led by single mothers who are living close to the poverty line.

4. The average married couple today has more parents than children.

5. Half of all marriages that began in the 1970s have ended or will end in divorce.

6. Single fathers are the fastest growing category of households: more than 1.4 million families. Although many are divorced, there is still another category of single fathers: never-married male heads of households.

7. Gay and lesbian couples now make up another fast-growing segment of the new family structure.

With these new family structures we need to be aware of how applicable our family assessment is and whom we need to include in both the medical and the psychosocial treatment plan. Never make assumptions about the composition of your patient's family.

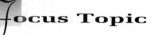

Focus Topic

The Impact of Breast-Feeding on Sexuality

Connie Tierno RN, MS Certified Lactation Consultant

> Suzanne is in a dilemma. She's 6 months pregnant and has been asked whether she will breast-feed or bottle-feed her baby. She's been reading a lot lately, and everything she's read says that human milk is the ideal food for human babies. She wants only the best for her baby, and she wants to be the best mother in the world. But how will Ron feel about a baby suckling at her breasts? He always thought of them as his. Will she be able to make love if milks leaks from her breasts? Will he find that repulsive? What about the baby? What does it feel like to have a baby nursing from your breasts? Does it hurt? Suzanne's breasts have always been rather sensitive. What if she feels sexually aroused? That would surely gross her out!

Not all women feel ambivalent about breast-feeding, but the above example depicts some of the issues that nursing a baby may unearth for the new mother. Although it is very difficult to make generalizations about this experience, both partners may harbor conflicting emotions related to breast-feeding and its effect on their sexual relationship.

In our Western culture, many young people have never even seen a baby nursing at its mother's breast. Breasts are viewed as sexual objects; their role in feeding and nurturing a baby is rarely acknowledged.

The nurse may need to suggest that the couple spend some time preparing for breast-feeding. Books and videos, classes, and support groups are available to the young couple contemplating this decision. It may also be helpful to encourage the couple to spend some time examining the breasts for nipple protrusion, and even occasionally massaging the breasts and expressing a drop or two of colostrum. These activities will help the couple begin to make the transition from thinking of the breasts as solely objects for sexual gratification. They can begin to discuss their feelings related to breast-feeding and their sexual relationship.

It is impossible to generalize, but breast-feeding may enhance or inhibit a couple's sexual relationship. For instance, some people feel that the lactating breasts are quite sensuous. Others may feel that breast milk spurting from the breasts during orgasm is a "mess." Mother may feel too exhausted by her responsibilities to her new baby to feel sexy. Father may feel jealous of the baby having unrestricted access to the breasts. Couples need to know that none of their feelings are right or wrong, but that it's important for them to find ways of expressing their love and concern for one another that are mutually satisfying.

If one or both partners are worried that breast-feeding may keep the father from getting to know his baby intimately, the nurse may suggest ways that he may develop a relationship with his baby. Bathing, massaging, cuddling, holding, and singing to the baby will all help to draw him closer to his child. When mother is breast-feeding, father can encircle his wife and baby in his arms or he can lie beside her as she feeds. When the baby is full, he can cuddle the baby up to his bare chest and rub his or her little back as they fall off to sleep together. Breast-feeding can be a shared experience.

Breast-feeding will not improve a poor sexual relationship anymore than having a child will improve a failing marriage. On the other hand, an already strong relationship can only be enhanced as the couple works together to bring their child into the circle of their love.

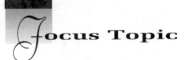

Focus Topic

Male Infertility

Infertility is a medical condition that can cause a great amount of anguish and pain for the couple who want to have a child. The drive to reproduce oneself seems to be one of the most powerful factors in our existence.

The criterion for infertility is usually defined as having unprotected intercourse for 1 year's time without becoming pregnant. In about 40% percent of infertility cases the problem lies with the female. In about another 40% the problem is with the male, and in the remaining 20% the fertility problem lies with both partners.

It has been estimated that as many as one out of five couples may be infertile. This rate rises with age. Increasingly we are finding that couples are delaying childbirth into their late 30s and 40s. Therefore, this problem seems to be occuring more often.

Little of the literature has focused upon the infertile man and the options available to him for conception. It seems that historically it was the "woman's" problem if conception did not occur or if the child was of the "wrong" sex. A glaring example of this attitude was Henry the VIII's quest for a male heir. Henry blamed the birth of his daughters on his wives and succeeded in divorcing or having them killed when they produced a female child.

Part of the myth and feelings regarding male sexuality is that men must be fertile to be successful sexually. Thus the male confronted with an infertility problem may feel that his sense of manliness and his self-esteem are challenged. These are issues that need to be sensitively handled.

Fortunately, we are becoming more and more successful in identifying and treating infertility. One way is through a sperm count. The male is asked to masturbate into a collecting cup, and the sperm are then counted. For the count to be considered fertile it must contain more than 20 million sperm/ml of semen. The leading cause of male infertility is a low sperm count.

The sperm will than be checked for normalcy, motility, and structure. It will also be checked to see if what has been ejaculated is considered to be within normal volume, which is 1 to 6 ml. A lab test will check to see if the semen has enough fructose (>1,200 µg/ml) to be viable.

If the sperm count is low, hormone levels of LH and adrogens will be checked in the blood or urine. The blood supply to the testes may also be checked. A sample of testicular tissue may be taken to see is spermatogenesis (the creation and the development of the sperm) is normal. Immunological tests to check whether the male is producing antibodies to his own sperm may also be evaluated and a physical exam may be performed to check the condition of the sex-accessory gland and ducts. As a result of the findings of the physical exam, one may be able to make the appropriate medical intervention so that 9 months later someone can happily assist the couple in the delivery room.

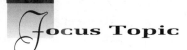

Focus Topic

Testicular Self-Exam

Cancer of the testes is a relatively rare form of cancer, accounting for approximately 1% of cancers in American men. The majority of these cancers occur in males between the ages of 20 to 44, which is typically the age when a man is most concerned about starting a family. Unfortunately, this cancer is frequently ignored, and rarely is it discussed by the public. If detected early before the cancer has spread to other parts of the body, testicular cancer can be completely cured nearly 100% of the time.

During the past 40 years the rate of this cancer for white men has nearly doubled and is now more than four times greater than among black men. A major risk factor is undescended testes. This condition is easily treated by surgery. Unfortunately, little boys are not always checked for this condition.

The most common finding leading to a diagnosis of testicular cancer is a hard lump, usually about the size of a pea. Other clinical signs include painless swelling in the testicle and a feeling of heaviness in the groin area or scrotum.

Men can help detect cancer of the testes in its earliest stages by practicing a simple technique known as *testicular self-examination (TSE)* every month. Ideally, this should be performed after a warm shower or bath, when the skin of the scrotum is relaxed, making it easier to feel anything unusual. In this exam, the man stands in front of a mirror and then gently rolls each testis between the thumb and fingers of both hands. (A booklet with more detailed instructions is available from the American Cancer Society.) If he feels anything unusual, he should notify his doctor. The technique is illustrated in Figure 5-1.

FIGURE 5—1
Testicular Self-Exam

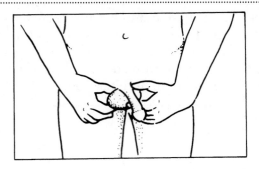 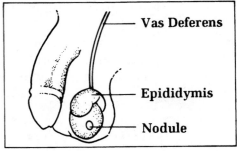

Vas Deferens

Epididymis

Nodule

Your best hope for early detection of testicular cancer is a simple three-minute monthly self-examination. The best time is after a warm bath or shower, when the scrotal skin is most relaxed.

Roll each testicle gently between the thumb and fingers of both hands. If you find any hard lumps or nodules, you should see your doctor promptly. They may not be malignant, but only your doctor can make the diagnosis.

Following a thorough physical examination, your doctor may perform certain x-ray studies to make the most accurate diagnosis possible.

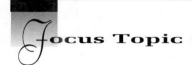

Focus Topic

Acquired Immunodeficiency Disease (AIDS)

By Al Rundio, Jr., RN, CNAA, CIC

Joe Doe is a 38-year-old single, white, bisexual male. Joe never considered himself to be promiscuous, however, he did have occasional receptive anal intercourse with different people. He always wondered whether he carried the AIDS virus. Friends of his had suggested on numerous occasions that "you are better off not knowing whether you are HIV positive or not." The thought of testing plagued Joe. Finally, one day he decided that he would see his family physician and ask him if he would order an HIV serum antibody test.

That Friday, Joe saw his physician. The ELISA test (electrophoresis immune serum assay), when checked twice, was positive for HIV. This, however, is not considered affirmation that one is carrying the AIDS virus. The laboratory performing Joe's HIV test then had to perform a western blot, another antibody test. If the western blot was positive, then Joe would know that he had been exposed to the HIV virus, but he would not know how infectious he was or whether he would go on to develop the full disease spectrum of AIDS.

Antibodies are developed by the body's immune system to ward off or fight any antigen that invades one's body. The antigen, which is usually a protein such as a bacteria or a virus is what actually causes the infection. Antibody testing merely states that the body has developed an immune response to an antigen. This response is specific. For example, the HIV antibody will not fight the measles virus; it will only work on the HIV virus. To really assess one's infectivity, antigen testing is needed. This will most likely be done in the very near future.

History and Facts

Joe is one of an estimated number of 1 to 2 million people in the United States who are infected with the human immunodeficiency virus, termed HIV. Since 1981, AIDS has plagued the United States. In 1982, gay men in San Francisco, Los Angeles, and New York City, began dying of bizarre opportunistic infections. The most common of these infections were pneumocystis carinii pneumonia (PCP) and Kaposi's sarcoma. PCP brought with it a dramatic increase in the number of requests to the Centers for Disease Control (CDC) for pentamidine, an experimental drug at the time which was used for treating PCP.

An investigation by the CDC, revealed that all the victims dying of these infections were gay men. Life-style investigation revealed that the average gay male with opportunistic infection had over 50 different sexual partners per year and an estimated 1,000-plus partners in a lifetime.

It was also discovered that many of these men used amyl nitrate or "poppers" to enhance sexual orgasm. Many or these victims also frequented venereal clinics for the treatment of gonorrhea, chlamydia, and syphilis. The disease killing these young men (the majority were in their early 20s and 30s) was first called GRID, which stood for gay-related infectious disease.

Theories suggested that the numerous sexual contacts, exposure to frequent bouts of sexually transmitted disease, and the use of amyl nitrates challenged one's immune system to the point that cellular immunity weakened, thus rendering the body prone to *opportunistic infection*. Microorganisms normally do not take advantage of a host with an intact immune system, even if they reside in the human's environment. However, when the immune system fails, these microorganisms take advantage or "opportunity" of the host.

There are several such organisms. The most common are cytomegalovirus or CMV, herpes simplex virus, Cryptococcus, Mycobacterium tuberculosis (the acid-fast organism that causes tuberculosis), Mycobacterium avium-intracellulare, Candida albicans (a fungus that causes thrush in newborns), and helminths (parasitic wormlike organisms in the intestines). Pneumocystis carinii pneumonia (PCP) and Kaposi's sarcoma (normally a very slow-growing cancer in elderly men of Mediterranean descent) are the most common diseases.

A few months after the CDC had coined the name of GRID for these young men, heterosexual women who abused intravenous drugs also began to die from the same opportunistic infections. The CDC then changed the name from GRIDS to AIDS, which stands for acquired immunodeficiency syndrome.

Researchers continued to work on the epidemic, which was growing at a phenomenal pace. The biggest fear was that statistics were going to spiral in the heterosexual population. In 1992, 9% of the victims infected with HIV were heterosexual.

In the mid-1980s, Montagnier, a French researcher at the Institute of Pasteur in Paris, France, discovered a virus that he believes causes AIDS. Six months later, in the United States, Robert Gallo also discovered this same virus.

What has been learned about the human immunodeficiency virus since its discovery? HIV is a retrovirus. The genetic core of HIV is RNA (ribonucleic acid). HIV is also an *intracellular virus*; that is, it enters the cell that it affects. It has an affinity for the T 4 helper cells which assist in priming one's immune system from within the cell in a process is known as cell-mediated immunity. HIV will actually change the genetic core, the DNA, of the T 4 helper cell and prevent this cell from functioning as an immune system cell. Rather, it will produce more budding viral particles of HIV, so that more infection can ensue in other T 4 helper cells. As T 4 helper cells are destroyed, the body's immunity begins to weaken, thus leaving the body open to opportunistic infection.

Transmission and Prognosis

It is believed that HIV is transmitted in several different ways. Although it is present in a majority of body fluids, the largest presence is found in the blood; hence, HIV is really a blood-borne organism. Thus, for the transmission of HIV, it only makes sense that some exchange of body fluid, in particular blood, must occur. The primary routes of transmission include the sharing of contaminated intravenous needles among drug addicts, receptive anal intercourse, heterosexual intercourse (although transmission seems less probable than with receptive anal intercourse), blood transfusion, and exchanges of blood products (factor B of hemophiliacs).

However, the majority of these blood products are now safe secondary to a heat-treating fractionalization process. Accidental mucous membrane splashing and needlestick incidents among health care workers has also decreased. The transmission rate today in health care workers is approximately 0.4%.

Once HIV was discovered, laboratories quickly worked on developing antibody tests. In 1985, these tests were available. The most important tests are the ELISA and the western blot, already mentioned. Since the ELISA has a 2% false negative and false positive rate, confirmation of HIV is made with the western blot test. Normal procedure is to do an ELISA test first. If this test is positive, a second ELISA test is performed. If this second ElISA test is positive, a western blot test is then performed to confirm or not confirm HIV seropositivity. All donated blood is now screened with the ELISA test. If the test is positive, the blood is discarded rather than risk the transmission of HIV.

There is much controversy over several aspects of AIDS today. Most scientists and researchers feel that once a person is infected with the HIV virus the probability of going on to develop full-blown AIDS is nearly 100%. However, using Karl Popper's refutation theory of science—that is, one must try to disprove a theory in order to truly validate it—a few scientists and researchers are of the opinion that one does not necessarily go on to develop full-blown AIDS even if infected with the HIV virus.

These AIDS theorists feel that AIDS is typical of any other infectious disease. As with any epidemic, some people become infected and die, others become infected and become ill but eventually recover, others never become ill but just develop an antibody to the organism, and others are not ill themselves but have subclinical infections and carry the disease organism. These last people can certainly transmit it to others.

Typhoid Mary is the best example of a subclinical infection. Although she was infected with the Salmonella type microorganism and certainly transmitted it to others (she worked in the kitchens of hospitals and killed whole wards of patients by transmitting the organism she was carrying), for some reason she herself never developed typhoid fever. The organism lived symbiotically with its host, Typhoid Mary. It is interesting to note that Typhoid Mary was quarantined on an island and died at age 76 of a stroke.

These same AIDS researchers stress that HIV is only one component of becoming ill with the disease syndrome known as AIDS. They are firm believers in the *cofactor theory*; that is, other cofactors must be present in order for one to develop full-blown AIDS. For example, frequent receptive anal intercourse may be one such cofactor. The Epstein-Barr virus may be another. The use of amyl nitrates as sexual stimulators may be another cofactor, and drug abuse itself may be a cofactor in the development of AIDS.

Some of these theorists also believe that if one removes one cofactor, such as by stopping receptive anal intercourse, the HIV antibody level will eventually drop and even disappear. Who is correct? We have yet to find this out. But one thing is quite evident: if the HIV virus were easily transmitted, then droves of people would have the disease. Thus it is extremely doubtful that HIV is transmitted casually. Even transmission through saliva has yet to be documented. A blood-to-blood exchange of body fluid seems necessary.

The best news is that HIV infection is totally preventable. Monogamy is stressed. Use of latex condoms with nonoxynol-9 (a spermicide that kills the HIV virus) is a must for sexually active people. Although not a 100% guarantee against AIDS, condoms are one effective mechanism of disease prevention.

Clean needle exchange programs for addicts warrants further exploration. And universal precautions for health care workers is mandatory. The best weapon that we have in our arsenal is education: we need to continually educate the public on disease prevention. Although vaccine development is progressing, this process is difficult because the HIV virus goes through what is known as an *antigenic drift*; that is its molecular structure changes. Flu epidemics occur for the same reason: flu vaccines do not work because the virus has already "drifted," or changed its structure by the time the vaccine is used. There is also the ethical question of vaccine trials. Who do we test the vaccine on? Would you elect to be a human subject?

Treatment of HIV infection varies. AZT, DDI, Zidovudine, DiDanosine, and combination therapy seem to have the best results. Although there is no cure for HIV infection, people are living longer with AIDS. Thus AIDS is really a chronic disease at the present time. Case fatality rates are actually declining as victims of this disease are now living longer. Nurses therefore need to consider the chronicity of HIV infection and AIDS rather than its acute aspect.

Nursing Interventions

What role does nursing play in caring for a patient with HIV infection? The best model for nursing is that of the nursing process: assessment, planning, intervention, and evaluation, and then repetition of this cycle. During an initial assessment, nurses must look at the whole picture; the patient deserves to be treated from a holistic perspective. Thus not only should nurses be concerned with the physical status of the patient and what opportunistic infections are apparent, but they must also pay strict attention to the psychosocial aspects of patient care.

Often, patients with HIV infection are not only facing the diagnosis of being HIV infected or having AIDS, but may also for the first time have to reveal their bisexuality, homosexuality, or whatever risk factor is apparent, to family or friends. Thus, they often lose their sexual privacy.

Concerns such as job security also become important. Thankfully, the U. S. government enacted federal legislation in 1992 that protects the patient with AIDS through the American Disabilities Act: AIDS is considered a disability. The CDC has also redefined its case definition for AIDS. A patient no longer has to have opportunistic infection to be labeled as having AIDS; low T 4 helper cell counts is the determining factor.

Nurses also need to look back over 100 years ago to the days of Florence Nightingale, the founder of modern nursing. Nightingale stressed the importance of the interaction of the environment and the patient. She was adamant about proper nutrition, clean air, and a healthy environment and life-style. Her theories do work. During the Crimean War, soldiers were dying by the droves. Nightingale's attention to a clean environment, proper waste disposal systems, and good nutrition as well as holistic patient care improved the outcomes of the men fighting in battle.

Along with giving holistic care, nurses must pay attention to the educational needs of each patient. Transmission of the virus and prevention of transmission should be stressed. How to live a healthy life-style needs to be emphasized, including stress reduction strategies. Guided imagery, meditation, hypnosis, and other nontraditional methods can be employed for the PWA (person with AIDS).

It is obvious that a certain number of patients will succumb to this disease process. Nursing's role then is to provide grief counseling to family members and to allow the patient to die with dignity.

Joe Doe remained AIDS free for several years. Although his HIV serum antibody status remained positive, Joe led a healthy life-style. This he attributed to the role that nursing played. Rather than looking only at germ theory—that is, fighting the HIV virus—nursing stressed the other factors in Joe's life—that is, what made him function as a human being. Treating Joe holistically may enable him to be a productive member of society for many years.

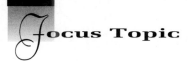

ocus Topic

An Overview of Early Adulthood

Object-relations theory: The developmental tasks of this stage include distancing oneself from family of origin, attachments and investments in a mate or significant others, and children and career.

Erikson/intimacy versus isolation: Young adults need to separate from their family of origin and begin to develop new relationships based on commitments related to sharing one's adult life. These relationships will create a new family for the young adult.

Tasks of this stage: Basic decision making regarding education, life mate, sharing of mutual intimacy in marriage or in other relationships; and life-style.

Sexuality: This is the stage of values. Sexual orientation becomes more consolidated. Challenges may be the first pregnancy, abortion, the first use of contraception or for some the first birth of a child, nursing, and planned parenthood.

Chapter 6

Smack in the Middle: Midlife

Laura was making an apple pie. All of her three children were coming home from college for Easter break. Although she was feeling happy to see them, she also had some mixed feelings about seeing her youngest daughter, Susan. It wasn't that she didn't love Susan. However, when Susan was home she tended to walk around as if she was still in her college dorm. Laura couldn't help but notice how full and large Susan's breasts were and how different her breasts were from Laura's.

Laura was waiting for a breast implant, and Susan's healthy breasts were a painful reminder and concern (breast cancer runs in her family). Laura kept on mixing the cake while thinking about simpler times and waiting for the doorbell to ring.

Midlife sexuality is not usually a topic that we are totally comfortable discussing. Imagine the discomfort for the midlife patient who has a sexual concern or has the potential for developing a sexual problem related to an illness. Imagine the intensity of this discomfort if the nurse or physician is 20 years younger than the patient. Developing a sensitivity to the physical and emotional vulnerabilities that may affect this age group is very important to be both effective and empathetic in their care.

CULTURAL ATTITUDES ABOUT MIDLIFE

These vulnerabilities and attitudes are further influenced by our culture, which highly values the young as sexual beings. Unlike some of the European cultures this attitude of youth worshipping is more exagerated in American culture. Unfortunately, the young are typically defined as those individuals under the age of 40. *Forty is equated with aging!*

If you are feeling skeptical of this statement, just turn on the television or the radio or open up a magazine to learn how you can remain looking young. How many of the models are over 40? The strongest message coming from the media is that lovemaking and sexuality are exclusively for the young and beautiful, single, and physically healthy. Contemporary America seems to be in love with the image of youth.

Within a historical context, the United States can be perceived as having evolved from a society that initially venerated the aged. The Puritan tradition, for example equated age with wisdom and spirituality. But today we can be perceived as a "throwaway" culture that venerates youth and/or youthful behavior.

With the advent of an industrial society, the positive status of the elderly changed as a result of several factors, including an increase in modern health technology which enabled many more people to grow old. Manual jobs were also replaced with high-technology positions that necessitated fewer people in the work force. The elderly therefore, became competition in terms of work positions. The loss of the extended family living together lowered the need for the elderly to be babysitters and helpers around the home, and the growth of literacy obviated the need for the aged to be the historians of the culture. The result of all this was *ageism*, or prejudice against the elderly.

As a result of ageism, there has been very little research on midlife sexuality. In fact, only one doctoral dissertation written in the past 100 years has specifically researched the sexual functioning of women during their midlife years. This was written by the author. I believe that many researchers are simply too uncomfortable with the concept of aging and sexuality to pursue the subject.

In addition, the few researchers who have studied sex and aging have found great reluctance among older people to discuss their sexuality. According to Goldman (1991), although everyone aspires to have a long life, it seems that no one wants to get older. Perhaps this conflicting desire may be the foundation of our basic prejudice against aging.

EXPECTATIONS ABOUT SEXUALITY

Expectations about sexuality and aging are basically culturally defined. In approximately 70% of the cultures that are in existence at the present time, the elderly continue to be sexually active. Although attitudes are slowly changing, in our Judaic-Christian culture the belief that the value of sex is primarily for procreation is still considered to be present for many groups within the culture. As a result, women past childbearing years are not acknowledged nor encouraged to be sexual.

In our society, the vast majority of people believe that sexual behavior declines with age. Since most parents keep their sexuality secret from their children, this myth along with these attitudes, becomes self-perpetuated with each new generation of younger people.

Sigmund Freud believed that witnessing parents having intercourse was traumatic to children and could even contribute to extreme pathology in adulthood. On a more humorous note, the late philosopher-humorist Sam Levinson stated the following when he first recalled finding out how babies were made: "To think my mother and father would do such a thing! My father, maybe; but my mother—never."

In this regard, society has dealt especially harshly with women. Being female, in midlife, and also confronted with the concept of being sexual has prompted ambivalence, confusion, discomfort, and ignorance in contemporary American culture. As a consequence, although there are now exceptions to the perpetuation, a cultural belief system exists that continues the myth that midlife women, even more so than men, are not interested in sexuality.

This is a tragedy, because there are approximately 32 million women between the ages of 40 and 65 in the United States. Contemporary attitudes regarding sexuality and aging in women have placed older women in a very disadvantaged environment. Furthermore, according to several sexologists, whatever cultural status women have is based almost entirely upon their sexuality. This is indeed "a double whammy."

These cultural attitudes are not experienced within a vacuum. Midlife men and women may well sense the attitudes of not only their own children but also that of the media and of the health professionals that care for them. Thus the implications for this ageist belief system are very important for nurses to recognize. When the average life expectancy was 47 years (circa 1900), we did not have to learn to feel comfortable about being sexual during midlife or old age. We did not have to adjust our self-concept toward a body that did not react with the same sexual "speed" as in our youth. Today, our patients hopefully have a much longer life expectancy, and they need professionals to help them remain sexual as they age.

To ensure sexual health, we need to be aware of the issues and concerns of the midlife patient. It is important to recognize that these concerns are also influenced by culture, religious beliefs, gender, and the psychological health of the client and of ourselves.

Another threat to the midlife woman and man is the emerging sexuality of their daughters and sons. Typically, men and women during midlife have children who are in their teen years. It may be threatening and confusing for middle-aged parents to be confronted with their own changes in self-image as their children reach sexual maturity. These existential issues can affect not only one's sense of well-being but also sexual expression.

DEVELOPMENTAL ISSUES OF MIDLIFE

As stated in the previous section, the concept of midlife is a relatively contemporary phenomenon, and the development of an accurate body of knowledge regarding the dynamics of this stage is in an exploratory stage. This knowledge is relevant for nursing because the developmental issues, experiences, and concerns of midlife patients will affect not only upon their experience of their illness but also their ability to be educated in health care.

Unfortunately, until the past decade, studies of adult development viewed the phase of midlife as a relatively static period between the ages of adolescence and old age. However, in the past two decades this analysis has changed, and middle age is beginning to be perceived as a time of development and growth.

Erik Erikson believed that the psychosocial task of midlife (stage seven) was resolving the conflict between *generativity versus stagnation or self-absorption*. Generativity implies the responsibility to take care of the family, and the society at large. It is a time of increasing integration with the larger world; the midlife individual may well be responsible for the leadership of society. Conversely, it may be a time of negativity, where the individuals begin to reassess their identity and their accomplishments and realize that the dreams they aspired to may not occur.

Gender and Midlife

However, it is very interesting to note that there is a new trend toward understanding human development in terms of gender. Feminist scholars argue that most studies of human development, such as those by Freud (1925), Erikson (1959) and Levinson (1986), have analyzed the experiences of women through the voices of men. They have therefore discounted the uniqueness of how women view themselves and their interaction with the society at large. The feminist literature believes that women experience a different time frame in the achievement of developmental issues such as identity and intimacy.

Neugarten has found that women, but not men, define their age status in terms of the timing of events within the family cycle. For example, unmarried career women in her study discussed middle age in terms of the family they might have had. Married women closely linked their sense of middle age to the launching of their children into the adult world.

In a review of the literature on midlife women, Lewitte (1982) emphasizes that there is general agreement that for women the midlife crisis centers around the diminishing or end of the reproductive role, rather than on biological change, or the realization that aging and death are inevitable. Another critical issue for women at midlife is the loss of attractiveness, or more correctly what the culture values as attractive: to look very young. Rubin believes that it is not aging itself but rather the fact that many women derive self-worth from their physical appeal to men that causes such turmoil.

What are the developmental sequences and concerns that women experience? There is a growing consensus, among feminist developmentalists that females, more so than males, are defined by their relation to other people, especially their families (Norman, 1979). Nancy Chodorow (1974), a psychotherapist, attributed the nearly universal differences between masculine and feminine personalities and roles to the fact that women are universally responsible for early child care. She felt that as a result of this experience boys and girls experience the early social environment differently and develop different basic personalities. She believed that the feminine personality, more so than the masculine personality, defines itself in the context of relationships.

This may be why we frequently see female family members and friends more comfortably supportive of their friends who are patients. It may also help to explain why so many more women are placed in the empathic role of nurse and caregiver. Gilligan, a feminist psychologist (1982) writes:

> Masculinity is defined through separation while femininity is defined through attachment. Male gender identity is threatened by intimacy while female gender identity is threatened by separation. Thus men tend to have difficulty with relationships, while females tend to have problems with individuation.

Gilligan (1982) theorizes that women's moral development centers around intimacy, relationships, and care, whereas for men it is based on a sense of "law and order." If this is true, these different experiences will certainly affect the self-perception of the male and female patient and how much neediness and dependency they allow themselves. The man who is now dependent on someone for all of his activities of daily living may need a great amount of psychological work to cope with these issues. The woman who has also been the primary caregiver for her family may find great difficulty in asking for help and letting down her family by becoming ill. When these sex roles become challenged, you may witness a great amount of chaos and confusion. Sex roles now need to become renegotiated and reevaluated, redefined and reorganized.

Barnett (1985) and Baruch et al. (1983) studied a group of almost 300 women between the ages of 35 to 55 to determine what factors contribute to women's healthy adjustment to the middle years. They concluded that certain elements influenced a woman's mental health. These were a woman's sense of mastery or control over her life and also how pleasurable she perceived her life to be. Neither criterion was correlated with age. Paid work was the single best predictor of mastery, and a positive experience with husband and children (including a good sex life) was the best predictor of pleasure.

The women that we see as patients may therefore be assumed to be going through a period of transition as they begin to define themselves not only in the context of family but also in terms of how satisfying other arenas of their life have been. Although men are also going through a midlife transition, their status and power may still be their focal point for reflection. However, I believe that this too is changing and that men are slowly becoming in touch with those attributes which foster the gentler, more expressive side of their personality. However, as nurses we need to be wary of making broad generalizations related to gender rather than to the individual.

Relationships

Another aspect of middle adulthood relates to changing relationship needs. For example, some men and women who were content to be single through their younger years now begin to question their prior choices and now want long-term commitment and relationships. For women this seems to be a more difficult task, since men have been given far more latitude in terms of dating than women. In our culture, men can date women older, younger, and the same age as themselves. Typically, women have not been given that same freedom: they are supposed to date men older than themselves. Furthermore, whereas the physical attractiveness of the man is frequently perceived to be of less importance than his power or prestige, for the middle-aged woman, in general, appearance is frequently considered to be of more importance if she is going to attract men. However, attitudes are slowly changing and we need to recognize the unique diversities of our patients.

Contrary to belief, divorce does not become more prevalent during middle age. In fact, most of the marriages that have lasted until middle age typically stay together even if they are not happy. However, for those marriages that are caught in an emotionless relationship sexual interest tends to wane.

Decreased sexual desire may occur as well as sexual dysfunctions. These may be experienced as the end result of pent up hostility toward the partner or even just sexual boredom. Extramarital affairs are also a possible reaction to marital apathy. With the advent of AIDS and fear of contracting the disease, however, extramarital affairs are not as common as in former times.

The Gay Population and Midlife

Another population that health professionals need to be aware of is the middle-age homosexual male or female. Like our patients in the heterosexual population, they have a variety of reactions to middle age. Some gay men in their 40s feel that they are not attractive enough to get younger men. Gay males who have previously led a life based on sexual conquests or being known for their sexual prowess will find this time a difficult transition. Similarly to heterosexual men, they may resort to facelifts or hair transplants to look younger. This is also the time during the life span when gay men who were previously married may more frequently "come out" and live a more openly gay lifestyle.

Middle age is also a time when parental influence and opinion is not as important as before. If parents have passed away, their grown children may no longer have the need to hide their sexual orientation. For many gay men, however, this is a period of existential crisis, especially if they continue to "hide" their sexuality.

It is important for nurses to recognize and understand that not every couple that we meet in the health care setting is heterosexual. Many are gay. We need to be aware of our preconceptions if we are going to relate successfully with our patients and their sexual concerns during an illness. One situation in which we may see many gay couples is when a partner comes into the health care setting with a diagnosis of AIDS. It is important to be sensitive to the needs and privacy of this couple as they go through what is typically a very traumatic event.

Indeed, throughout the 1990s the nurse professional will probably see significant changes in the way that both males and females view themselves and their roles in society as a whole. In fact, the nurse too, may also see attitudal changes in him or herself related to their own sense of self. The sexual issues of the midlife patient may engender many challenges on the emotional and intellectual capabilities of the nurse as a caregiver.

PHYSICAL CHANGES

As we age certain physical changes occur that can affect our appearance, our health, and our sexuality. For both men and women middle age is usually a time when physical functioning and health are still good, although not at the peak of early adulthood.

Overt physical changes do begin to occur, however, including the graying of hair and loss of hair and teeth. The ears and the nose may become elongated. There may be subcutaneous fat losses and additional skin wrinkles. Eyesight and hearing may fail. Postural changes and a progressive structural decline may eventually result in a shortened trunk with comparatively long arms and legs.

However, the truism of "use it or lose it" seems to hold true for physical endurance. Those people of middle age who maintain their physical shape through exercise are typically in better health as they age.

The biological determinants that affect sexual functioning also begin to produce physiological changes during midlife. These changes are reviewed in the following section. To have a greater understanding of this material, it may be helpful to review the chapter on the sexual anatomy and the sexual response cycle. Throughout this discussion it is important to remember that aging alone does not diminish female or male sexual interest or the potential to enjoy sexuality.

Changes in Women

The sexual response of women in midlife changes in a number of body systems and organs. These include the breasts, muscles, clitoris, outer labia, inner labia, Bartholin's gland, and the vagina. In the breasts dense glandular tissue is replaced by fat and thus the breasts begin to sag. General muscle tone decreases with age. There is a loss of fatty-tissue deposits in the face and body.

Vaginal changes also occur. There is a decrease of elasticity and fullness in the vagina. The clitoris slowly atrophies and the major and minor labia no longer flatten. The expansion of the inner two-thirds of the vagina that typically occurs in younger women is slower to occur in older women. Vasocongestion of the outer third of the vagina is also reduced, although orgasmic tenting still occurs.

Lubrication of the vagina is controlled by the Bartholin gland, which secretes mucus during sexual stimulation. The secretory activity and quantity of this mucus appear to slow with aging, and after the age of 70 this secretion is nonevident. This condition can cause "painful intercourse" or *dyspareunia* because of severe dryness. Dyspareunia can frequently be treated with an artificial lubricant such as K-Y Jelly or Replens.

It has been found that women who are more sexually active seem to have more vaginal lubrication. Thus sexual activity may provide some protection against the normal aging changes in female anatomy and physiology.

Changes in Men

Sexual response in the male also slows down. This response is also a multisystem involvement that includes not only the sexual organs but also contributing parts of the body such as the muscular and vascular systems.

However, unlike women, who experience the end of their fertility as they reach 50, men do not necessarily become infertile. Indeed, there are reports of men in their late 70s and 80s who have fathered children. Sperm production does slow down after the age of 40. Although testosterone begins to decline as men age, men do not usually experience the major drops in hormones that women experience as they reach menopause.

As with women, however, the physiology of the sexual response in men is affected by aging in many ways. These changes, according to Masters and Johnson (1966), are the following:

1. Erection is a little harder to develop. It usually takes longer to get an erection and more direct stimulation of the penis is needed to achieve it. In younger men erection happens almost spontaneously.

2. Erections are not as firm as in a young man.

3. The testes (located in the scrotum) elevate only part way up to the perineum. They also do so more slowly than in younger men.

4. The amount of semen (fluid from the penis) is reduced, and the intensity of ejaculation ("come") is less.

5. There is usually less of a physical need to ejaculate. There is also absence of preejaculatory "seeping." Although a "dry" ejaculation is painful for older men, it is not as painful as with younger men.

6. The refractory period (time after orgasm and ejaculation, when the man is unable to ejaculate again) becomes much longer.

7. The sex flush does not usually occur in aging men. Muscle tension during sexual arousal is reduced as a result of reduced muscle strength and mass.

8. Sensations become less genital and may be more sensuous and diffused.

Implications for Nursing

All of the above changes can cause a great amount of anxiety to patients and their significant others if they are not aware that these changes are part of the normal physiological process that occurs as we get older. It has been the author's experience that this lack of knowledge may cause the couple not only to shut down sexually but even to dissolve a relationship. Frequently, partners will react to the slowing of the sexual response cycle with the projection that their mate no longer cares for them or that they are indeed undesirable. Unfortunately, I have seen worst-case scenarios in which a partner may even be accused of having an affair because the mate is not reacting with the same sexual intensity as before.

What can the health care professional do? It is paramount, first of all, to give patients permission to talk about their concerns regarding sexuality. We also need to educate them about the biology of aging and help them accommodate to these changes from both a psychological and physical perspective.

Nurses are a small microculture that reflects the mores or belief systems of the society at large. However, because we are viewed as professionals, we hold a large amount of power and prestige, and can use this power to educate patients. Many different books are available that can help patients address the myths and the concurrent feelings that they experience as they age. Bibliotherapy is an excellent tool for addressing these issues, not only for the patient but also for ourselves.

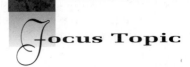

*F*ocus Topic

Breast Self-Exam

One out of nine women is expected to get breast cancer sometime during her life. This statistic has risen sharply in the past 10 years. We are not sure of the reason for this rise; however, there are certain facts that we do know about breast cancer.

Breast cancer is more likely to occur after the age of 40, and its risk increase sharply in the sixth and seventh decades of life. Risk factors include nulliparity, prolonged hormonal stimulation caused by early menses or a late onset of menopause, being of northern European descent, and having a first child after the age of 35. Other risk factors include having other cancers and being genetically predisposed to cancer. If a mother, sister, or aunt had or has breast cancer, the risk factor strongly rises. There have been no significant studies linking birth control pills or hormonal replacement therapy with breast cancer.

One of the most important health behaviors a woman can practice is monthly breast self-exam (BSE). It certainly is within the scope of nurses to advocate and teach BSE to their patients. There are numerous teaching charts and health aids available to help with patient teaching.

Breast self-exam should be done monthly. The best time of the month is after a woman has menstruated. If a women is in menopause, she should pick the same day every month so that she will remember to practice BSE. A good hint is to tell women to pick the same day as their birthday.

The best place for this exam is in the shower because it is easier to feel for any lumps when the skin is wet and soapy. There are several different techniques that can be used to examine the breasts. Figure 6-1 will be a helpful aid.

FIGURE 6–1
Breast Self-Exam

1. Lie down and put a pillow under your right shoulder. Place your right arm behind your head.

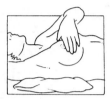

2. Use the finger pads of your three middle fingers on your left hand to feel for lumps or thickening. Your finger pads are the top third of each finger.

 Finger Pads

3. Press firmly enough to know how your breast feels. If you're not sure how hard to press, ask your health care provider. Or try to copy the way your health care provider uses the finger pads during a breast exam. Learn what your breast feels like most of the time. A firm ridge in the lower curve of each breast is normal.

4. Move around the breast in a set way. You can choose either the circle (A), the up and down line (B), or the wedge (C). Do it the same way every time. It will help you to make sure that you've gone over the entire breast area, and to remember how your breast feels.

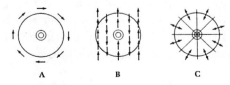

5. Now examine your left breast using right hand finger pads.

6. If you find any changes, see your doctor right away.

FIGURE 6–1 (continued)
Breast Self-Exam

You should also check your breasts while standing in front of a mirror right after you do your breast self-exam each month. See if there are any changes in the way your breasts look: dimpling of the skin, changes in the nipple, or redness or swelling.

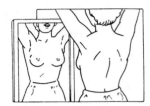

You might also want to do a breast self-exam while you're in the shower. Your soapy hands will glide over the wet skin making it easy to check how your breasts feel.

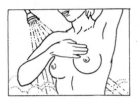

Used by permission. ©1992 American Cancer Society, Inc. Atlanta, GA. *How to do Breast Self Examination.*

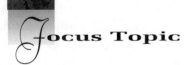

ocus Topic

Menopause

The menstrual cycles of women near the age of 50 become shorter, oligomenorrhea (lack of having a period) is more common, and fertility becomes lower as women stop ovulating. Eventually, women cease to menstruate. This is called *menopause.*

THE BIOLOGY OF MENOPAUSE

Menopause is the natural result of age-related changes in ovarian function. The word itself means "the cessation of uterine menstrual cycles."

Menopause occurs between the ages of 48 and 52. However, the changes that typically precede menopause begin for many women in their late 30s. This period of time is called the *perimenopausal period*. During the perimenopausal years the ovaries slowly begin to produce less estrogen. Many women patients experience menstrual irregularities such as heavy bleeding or irregular periods.

What causes menopause? One theory is that the ovaries cease to respond to FSH (follicule-stimulating hormone) and LH (luteinizing hormone) during the feedback loop. The feedback loop is a biological phenomenon when production of a product either increases or decreases further production of that product. In this case the feedback loop includes the pituitary gland and the ovaries. As discussed earlier, these two hormones are secreted from the pituitary gland, also known as the master gland. This lack of response is believed to be caused by a decrease in the blood supply in the ovaries.

Another theory of menopause is that the menses cease as a result of the exhaustion of the primary follicles. As women age, the ovarian follicles disintegrate. These are the follicles (approximately 500,000) that little girls are born with and that are found within the two ovaries.

In summary, during the period of peri- and postmenopause, women experience a significant change in their hormonal status. This change also influences other physiological symptoms. The most frequently reported cause of distress in perimenopausal women are vasomotor symptoms such as hot flashes, which bring on intense feelings of warmth in the skin (especially around the face) and profuse sweating. These hot flashes are caused by dilation of blood vessels in the skin, which bring in warm blood to these regions. The frequency of hot flashes varies. In extreme cases they can occur as often as every 10 minutes during the day or night. However, most women experience them much less frequently.

Other related symptoms that commonly occur during this period include dizziness, nausea, headaches, and night sweats. Approximately 75 to 85% of women experience some of these symptoms as they go through menopause.

A second symptom group directly linked to estrogen depletion is genitourinary atrophy. The epithelium of the vagina thins and loses rugal folds. A loss of elasticity leads to a decrease in vaginal depth. Vaginal fluid also decreases. Atrophy also occurs in the urethra. This may often cause urinary difficulties such as urinary tract and yeast infections. Chronic inflammation of the urethra is called urethritis.

Other physical signs of menopause may include shrinking of the external genitalia, the breasts, and the uterus. Women have also been reported to have signs and symptoms of peripheral neuropathy: numbness, itching, and clothing intolerance.

Some women may also gain weight. Fat frequently accumulates around the abdomen. Other symptoms include wrinkled skin, a deeper voice, and more facial hair. All of these changes can also cause psychological distress related to feelings about body image.

Another health concern is related to the potential for osteoporosis, the condition in which large amounts of calcium and phosphorus are lost from the bones. Osteoporosis places older women at high risk for broken bones, especially hips. Women also may lose height because of vertebrae compression. However, it is important to understand that not all women experience these physical symptoms, or if they do, they do not necessarily have to be of great intensity. Risk factors for osteoporosis include the following:

Family history of osteoporosis.

Reduced weight for height: very thin women are at higher risk.

Early menopause: before 48 years of age.

Low calcium intake: minimum of 500 mg. of calcium is needed daily.

Caucasian descent: especially light-skinned, northern European women.

Nulliparity.

Breast-feeding mothers who did not take a dietary calcium or supplement of calcium daily. This should be at least 2,000 mg daily.

High meat intake.

High alcohol intake.

High caffeine intake

Smoking.

Lack of physical activity: especially non-weight-bearing exercise.

Psychological Issues

Menopause can be a time of significant psychological adjustment. Some women need to sleep more: other women develop insomnia (sleep disturbances). Some women also experience a sense of loss when they no longer have their periods.

For women who have equated their femininity with fertility, the advent of menopause can strongly threaten their sense of not only their body image but also their sense of self. If this occurs at a time of other losses, such as parents dying or children leaving home, they may feel very vulnerable and may become depressed. For some women menopause is a negative reminder that they are aging and therefore coming closer to what may be perceived as the end of the life cycle. In our culture, with its emphasis on youth as the most desirable state of being, menopause may necessitate a major adjustment.

Sexuality

As these emotional experiences are occurring, some women experience lack of desire or other sexual problems. Menopause seems to produce a decline in sexual functioning, a decrease in level of sexual activity, a decrease in frequency of orgasm, and a decrease in vaginal lubrication. Although there are many theories related to this decrease in sexual activity it is not known whether these changes are the result of vaginal atrophy or lack of vaginal lubrication, which causes dyspareunia. Lack of lubrication, which causes painful intercourse, may also lead to less desire for sex and sexual activity. Estrogen deficiency may also have a direct impact on desire, arousability, and/or orgasmic capability.

Implications for Nursing

All of the above symptoms and changes in a woman's body can trigger both physical and emotional reactions. One of the empowering ways that we can make helpful interventions is through education and counseling. This should include not only the woman but also, if she is in a relationship, her significant other. Both women and men need to understand the changes that occur during the aging process. If they remain ignorant, they run the risk of endangering not only their physical and mental health, but also their relationships.

It is important to also be aware of the history that women bring with them. What were the messages and beliefs that the woman's family held regarding menopause? How did her mother experience and behave during menopause? What messages did the women in her family give her?

What were her experiences with older relatives or friends who had finished menopause? Is she anticipating "problems"?

Physical assessment is also important. The nurse should consider the type of period the woman is experiencing and if there is heavy blood loss. Information regarding diet, relaxation, vitamins, and important life-style changes may be beneficial. These may include the use of relaxation, exercise, and other holistic modalities.

Another frequent intervention is estrogen replacement therapy. For many years there have been medical debates regarding the safety and effectiveness of using *hormone replacement therapy (HRT)* during menopause.

Originally estrogen alone was effectively used to treat the symptoms of menopause. However, studies showed that there was a 4 to 13 times greater incidence of uterine cancer in these women. Estrogen was then combined with progesterone (which biologically has some antiestrogen properties). The combined used of *both* estrogen and progesterone does not cause an increase in the incidence of uterine cancer.

Today, various treatment cycles are used. The most common regimen is taking estrogen from the 1st day of the month through the 25th day and taking progesterone from the 16th day of the month through the 25th day. This dosage pattern closely mimics the hormone activity of a woman's naturally occurring menstrual cycle.

Hormone replacement therapy seems to be the most effective way of responding to the menopausal symptoms of hot flashes and night sweats. Other symptoms that frequently respond to HRT are memory impairment, depression, irritability, vaginal dryness, urinary frequency, and urge incontinence.

Finally, there is no indication that this kind of hormone replacement therapy increases the rate of breast cancer. However, HRT is absolutely contraindicated if there has been previous breast carcinoma, endometrial carcinoma, and endometrial hyperplasia. Other medical conditions that warrant weighing the benefits versus the risk factors of HRT include previous heart attack, previous stroke, abnormal blood lipids (fats), thromboembolic disease, breast dysplasia, acute liver disease, obesity, heavy smoking, estrogen-dependent pelvic disease such as fibroids, and a strong family history of breast cancer.

Estrogen also appears to play a protective role in preventing coronary heart disease and the bone loss involved in osteoporosis. The risk of developing breast or endometrial cancer as a result of taking HRT has also been basically disproven. HRT has also been found to help alleviate vasomotor discomfort and atrophic vaginitis.

At the present time, the role of estrogen in maintaining normal sexual function is still unclear. Many variables have clouded the issue of its effectiveness. These have included whether a woman has undergone a surgical or natural menopause and the number of years that she has been menopausal. However, considering the fact that women can expect to live almost 30 years after menopause, the benefits derived from using HRT, not only for maintaining sexual functioning but also for physical comfort, seem to be significant.

Pregnancy can sometimes still occur during the transition into menopause. It is therefore important to have your patient use some form of protection until there is little doubt of the possibility of becoming pregnant. Unfortunately, when pregnancy does occur, women are at a higher risk of having a baby who may have Down's syndrome.

Nurses can help women experience menopause in a nontraumatic manner by being supportive of their feelings and giving them permission to discuss their feelings and concerns. One very helpful intervention is a menopause support group where men and women can have a safe place to share their experiences and feelings.

Since we do not dispute the mind-body connection, it is important to consider all of the suggestions that have been discussed. Menopause should not be as traumatic as it has been for some women and their spouses or significant others. We can make a difference.

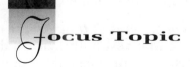

Focus Topic

Reading List for Midlife Sexuality

There are many helpful books available through bookstores and the library that you can suggest for your patients. A list of some of these books follows:

SUGGESTED READING

Butler, R. N. & Lewis, M. *Love and sex after forty/midlife.* New York: Harper and Row, 1986.

Doress, P. *Ourselves, growing older: Women aging with knowledge and power.* New York: Simon and Schuster, 1987.

Greenwood, S. *Menopause, naturally: Preparing for the second half of life.* San Francisco: Volcano, 1989.

Kahn, A. P. *Midlife health: A woman's practical guide to feeling good.* New York: Avon Books, 1987.

Lark, S. *The Menopause Self-Help Book: A Woman's Guide to Feeling Wonderful For the Second Half of Her Life.* CA: Celestial Arts, 1990.

Reitz, R. *Menopause: A positive approach.* Radnor, PA: 1977.

Schover, L. *Prime time: Sexual health for men over | 336 fty.* New York: Holt, Rinehart and Winston, 1984.

Voda, A. M., Dinnerstein, M., and & O' Donnell, S. (eds). *Changing perspectives on menopause.* Univ. of Texas Press, 1992.

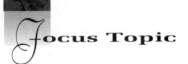

ocus Topic

Midlife Overview

Object-relations theory: There may be increased connectiveness with the family of origin. Adults learn to compensate for disappointments. Often there is a sense of emotional levelness and balance.

Erikson/Generativity versus stagnation or self-absorption: Adults must develop an "other"-focused philosophy and invest in the care of the world. Generative behaviors include assuming responsibility for a family, society, education, civic affairs, and social issues.

Stage in family life cycle: Families may have young, adolescent, or older children.

Tasks of this stage: Parenting, continued intimacy, becoming more competent in terms of career, being the sandwich generation (caring for children and parents concurrently), grandparenting, returning to school. For women, developing a new independence as the children leave home is important.

Sexuality: Menopause for women may end the childbearing years. Sexual expression versus sexual performance becomes an issue as the sexual response cycle becomes slower. Other issues are hormonal therapy, voluntary sterilization, new sex roles for men and women who have not had children, threats to body image in terms of getting older, coping with adolescents', emerging sexuality, remaining in relationships, midlife crisis.

Stressors related to illness: Parental responsibilities, aging parents, body image threats, advent of chronic disease and the need to adjust to this, changing roles in the family or relationship, finances, sense of mortality.

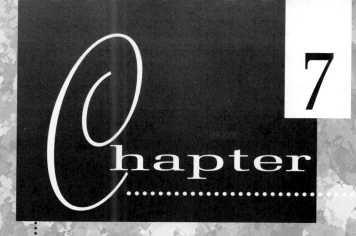

Chapter 7

Sexuality
and Aging

Every time that he saw her his heart would begin to race. He tried to make very clever, intelligent conversations with her or to those around her so that she might think that he was exciting and interesting. He noticed and thought about the way that she smiled and her funny little laugh. Around her he felt young and a little bit carefree, just how it had been 40 years ago when he had first fallen in love with his wife Annie. He missed his wife. But she had passed away almost 3 years ago. When he talked to Janice, some of the pain of Annie's death seemed to be less poignant. He was really looking forward to his birthday date this Friday. What better way to spend your 80th birthday than with an exciting, sensual woman!

Sexuality exists in various forms throughout the life cycle. However, the need for sexual expression exists for most individuals throughout their entire life span.

AGEISM

Ageism has existed throughout history. Unfortunately, ageism can be very destructive toward the sexual expression of the elderly. The older the patient, the more likely that ageist feelings will exist in our culture. Although ageism also exists toward the middle-age patient, it is typically more prevalent and frequently more overtly directed toward the older patient.

Recent studies have challenged ageist beliefs regarding sexuality and the reality of what is sexual behavior in the elderly. The most commonly held myth is that the elderly are asexual. What these studies are finding is that there is a stability in levels of sexual activity and capacity from about the age of 40 to the end of life. The keys to maintaining this sexual stability are felt to be good health and a cooperative partner. The most important motivators for continued sexual expression seem to be past interest in sex as young and middle-aged adults.

Frequently these ageist attitudes negatively influence our older patients. Expectations about sexuality in the later years are somewhat culturally defined and sexual behavior in the elderly is related to cultural expectations. In fact, in over 70% of the societies studied worldwide, the elderly continued to be sexually active. However, these are the societies where the elderly *are expected to be* sexually active. The prevalent view of our society is that older people are not sexual. As a result, many older patients are embarrassed to acknowledge their sexuality and therefore may not discuss their sexual concerns with you.

An interesting historical example reflecting our ageist belief system is given by Shakespeare's *Hamlet*, written almost 400 years ago. Hamlet epitomizes our culture's negative beliefs regarding getting older and being interested in sex. He says to his mother, Queen Gertrude: "At your age, the hey-day in the blood is tame." Hamlet could not begin to understand why his mother married with such "indecent haste" after his father's death. He denied that a woman of his mother's age could be motivated by love or passion. According to literary scholars who have studied Shakespeare's plays, Gertrude's age was probably less than 45.

ATTITUDES TOWARD SEXUAL EXPRESSION

There are many reasons why people have sex or are sexual, sexuality basically has two purposes: procreation and recreation. Although religious and cultural attitudes are slowly changing, following the decline of procreational ability (typically after menopause for women) our Judaic-Christian culture, as discussed in Chapter 2, frequently seems to deny or be uncomfortable with the role of the recreational or pleasurable aspects of sex. This attitude is especially true toward women past childbearing years. The image of older parentlike figures being sexual seems to cause a great amount of anxiety for younger people. As a consequence, one of the most uncomfortable topics for younger health professionals is the sexuality of the older patient.

Actually, it is my experience that sexuality is rarely addressed with any comfort to the older patient by any health professional. Possibly in reaction to our own discomfort, this topic is frequently treated with laughter and/or amusement. As a result, in spite of the increasing focus within the past 10 or 15 years on disseminating information regarding sexuality and sexual health, only brief consideration has been given to the sexuality of the aging.

This is very unfortunate. We now understand that sexual attitudes can affect a patient's mental, social, and physical self-image. Patients' sense of status as valued people in our society can be negatively affected by ageist attitudes. Generations of older people who have enjoyed sexuality and who consider it a pleasurable experience, may begin to question their "normalcy" in enjoying sex. Occasionally they may even become asexual as a result of our youth-oriented culture and our ageist ideas regarding who is entitled to be sexual. Older patients frequently feel embarrassed that they still enjoy sex! I have heard young nurses and physicians say, "Imagine! She's interested in having sex. Why, she is old enough to be my mother or grandmother." These professionals can obviously influence their older patients' sexual expression in a negative and destructive way.

According to the Bureau of the Census, as of 1989 there were 25.5 million Americans alive over the age of 65. This translates into one out of every nine persons in the United States. Few health professionals would deny the importance of helping these older adults achieve the highest quality of life possible, and this should include sexuality.

THE EXPERIENCE OF LOSS AND AGING

Erikson believed that the issue involved in this eighth stage of life is *integrity versus despair*. That is, the person needs to look back upon life and feel comfortable and satisfied with what has been achieved rather than feel that his or her life had no meaning and was riddled only with failure.

Aging is a difficult time during the life cycle because it is frequently filled with losses. Although we may experience losses throughout the life cycle it is in the aging population where they become prevalent. Unquestionably, loss is one of the most severe stressors that can affect our well-being and sexuality.

Loss of Significant Others

Loss is often caused by death, relocation, or simply the withdrawal of significant people in one's life. These may include spouses, significant others, children, friends, business associates, and friends.

Women are typically more at risk than men for experiencing loss as a result of death because statistics show that most women marry a man who is approximately 4 years older than themselves. Since a man's life expectancy is shorter than a woman's, the average woman is frequently a widow for 6 to 7 years after the death of her spouse. In the ninth decade and above there are approximately four women alive for every man. Frequently these women are not as physically independent as younger women, and the loss of independence as well as isolation, and poor health can cause major depression. Adjusting to living alone, without any appropriate modes of physical expression or social or physical connection, can be both frightening and depressing.

Loss of Cognitive Functioning

Although cognitive loss does occur for some, it seems to be less common among the elderly than has been assumed. Good nutrition may increase cognitive function. The increasing political power of the elderly also allows for more opportunities to participate in social and activist activities and not become disengaged and isolated. Being involved in the world discourages depression and its concurrent effect on cognition or thought processes. However, some of our patients may be cognitively impaired because of physical illness.

Another kind of physical loss that may occur is related to the diminishing strength of the five senses: seeing, hearing, smelling, tasting, and feeling. This decline can also contribute to cognitive confusion, emotional relatedness, and ability to be sexually expressive.

Loss of Role and Status

Western society measures self-worth by individual productivity and power; therefore, the loss of role typically causes a loss of status. Retirement still seems to affect males more negatively than females. However, in future generations, as more and more women seek professional careers, this issue will likely become of equal importance for both men and woman.

With retirement there are typically other related losses. These include lack of access to business friends, change in routine, lower status, and lower income capabilities. Time frequently becomes a burden as the loss of employment becomes an existential crisis creating questions related to the meaning of life and to an individual's self-worth. If employment gave professional satisfaction, the loss of that creative process may be felt.

Women may experience a different kind of loss when their spouses retire. If they now have a husband who is at home full-time, they may be forced to give up their women friends and become a more full-time companion to their spouse. They may also lose their independence and freedom in managing their homes. Couples with prior poor communication skills may find retirement especially difficult.

Thus retirement creates lifestyle changes for both men and women. These changes may influence the couple negatively, especially if the relationship was poor before retirement. New sets of role expectations will need to be negotiated and marital distress is common at this stage of life. However, in some couples retirement is a positive experience:

the couple welcomes this time to finally enjoy one another's companionship.

Women, more than men, may also perceive a loss of power caused by body image changes. When these changes are felt to reflect their desirability as sexual beings, they may experience profound feelings of grief and sadness.

Are men and women perceived differently as they age? Is growing older a different experience for men than for women? According to the feminist sociologist Sontag, the social belief that aging enhances a man's power but destroys women's power is perpetuated by women themselves. Sontag believes that our culture socially and sexually disenfranchises women as they age, and that Western societies feel condescending to the values and attributes of maturity. She also believes that society is more permissive about aging in men. According to Sontag, being physically attractive is more important in a woman's life because female beauty is identified with not only youthfulness but also with sense of worth.

Sontag describes one discomforting example of how a woman's terror may be symbolized: the statue created by the sculptor Rodin called Old Age. Old Age is a statue of a seated, naked old woman who is pathetically contemplating her flat, pendulous, ruined body. Sontag believes that biological aging in women is considered a cultural obscenity in our youth-oriented culture. The flabby bosom, wrinkled neck, and spotted hands, which are all signs of normal biological aging, are considered to be obscene by our cutural standards.

Thus, getting older for women, as already mentioned, seems to be a "double whammy." Women must cope with ageist stereotypes regarding their sexuality and attractiveness and also with increased body image changes such as wrinkling, age spots, and gray hair. They may also be facing instrumental body image changes related to medical problems such as hysterectomy and mastectomy.

Loss of Physical Power and Health

Approximately 86% of the elderly are believed to have at least one chronic disease which affects some part of their physical functioning. However, in 67% of this population there is no effect on mobility, and another 14% have no disability at all. So it may be safe to assume that a large number of the elderly are functioning very well. However, their health is typically not as good as that of younger men and women. In spite of the optimistic data just presented, the elderly do have more admissions to the hospital and do spend more time and energy coping with the advent of chronic illness. This can also create its own set of losses. These may include loss of mobility and increased pain, loss of energy and stamina, loss of body parts and their functions, and assaults to body image.

If depression occurs this frequently will decrease sexual desire. It is not true, however, that all members of this age group are depressed. For some, the lack of responsibility of caring for children and aging parents may be a welcome relief. For some older members of our culture aging is a positive and reflective time characterized by increased spirituality and acceptance.

Implications for Nursing

All of the above issues relate to patients' sense of well-being and consequently to their sexuality. When we meet with patients, it is important to look at, and discuss with them, their own loss history. This history affects the way that they feel, function, and interact with one another. This conversation will also help reinforce your acknowledgment of the deep losses that they may have suffered.

A glaring and common example of loss is exemplified by the widow who does not have a mate or sufficient opportunities to find a significant other sexual partner. If the older woman was culturally raised to believe that it is "wrong" to seek another mate, this may place her at even higher risk for not only becoming asexual but also becoming even more lonely and isolated. Unfortunately, many older men and women become disengaged from life as more of the people that were important to them either pass away or are geographically separated from them. It is extremely important for us to be sensitive to these loss issues.

When nurses interview an older patient, similarly to the younger patient they should include a sexual history. Again, we need to be aware of the feelings that this may trigger in ourselves as we interview the patient. If these feelings are too negative or will be destructive to the patient's sense of self, it is important to find another colleague to conduct the sexual history.

One important subject that should be included in the sexual history is masturbation. In some cultures and religions it is believed that masturbation is an unhealthy and unnatural act. However, autoerotic sexual activity is an important sexual outlet for the elderly and may actually increase in frequency as people age. In the nursing home, sexual intercourse is frequently not allowed, and masturbation may therefore be the only possible sexual activity there. Since it is an important outlet for experiencing sexuality, it should be discussed with these patients, especially if they believe that masturbation is bad or have never been given the opportunity to discuss their feelings regarding masterbation. Sometimes just giving patients bibliographic material discussing such sensitive subjects is very helpful in breaking down some of the sexual boundaries.

Losses in sexual functioning related to health issues are another necessary area to explore. This is important because frequently the myths related to aging become mixed up with the problems of chronic disease and/or depression. Patients who do not have correct information to understand what is related to illness and what is related to aging will not know how to make intelligent decisions. Many patients will just turn off their sexuality and never try to access the parts of their sexual functioning that are still available.

Another area for nurses to consider is grieving. For many of the aged, the death of a spouse symbolizes the end of sexual expression. Since older patients feel guilty if they seek another partner. It is important to discuss with patients normal grief. Facilitating a conversation that encourages them to understand how they are coping with this death may allow them to grieve in a positive and helpful way. This discussion may also help them determine what their emotional and sexual needs may be. Helping patients realize that finding another person for companionship or intimacy is normal and acceptable may be a constructive and necessary intervention.

Information related to how much information patients have regarding sexuality should be discussed, as well as the accuracy of that information. A discussion should also include feelings regarding themselves as sexual beings as they age. Our older patients may also be ageist. These are sensitive issues, and it may take time to develop comfort in discussing not only sexuality but also loss in your patients' lives. If we as nurses are successful in developing this degree of comfort, may certainly enhance our effectiveness in helping our aging patients.

SEXUAL INTEREST

There is a paucity of research on sexual functioning or dysfunction in the elderly. However, when older couples do cease sexual activity, the choice usually rests with disinterest or unavailability of a male partner. The earliest research on geriatric sexuality was done by Kinsey et al. (1948). Kinsey reported on the sexual histories of 106 men over the age of 60. This number is extremely small considering the fact that his survey included 14,000 males. Kinsey found that males were the most sexual active during late adolescence and that at age 60, four out of five men were capable of sexual intercourse. At the age of 80, only one man out four was capable of intercourse. Kinsey also found that sexual activity declined from two to three times a week at age 20, to .5 times a week at age 60.

Kinsey's investigations of sexual functioning in women also found a decline in sexual activity with aging. Women showed lower levels of sexual activity than men. These differences were related to marital status: that is, married women were significantly more sexually active than unmarried women. Thus, unavailability, not lack of interest of a partner seemed to be the most significant factor related to sexual functioning for women.

Masters and Johnson (1966) also emphasized the fact that the actual level of sexual interest in the aging individual was related to lifelong interest and activity. They believed that these changes would be less traumatic if they could be accepted and understood. Women, according to Masters and Johnson (1966), showed less change in interest as they age.

The Duke University longitudinal study (1960—1972) (Pfeiffer 1968) is considered the most ambitious study of aging and sexuality. This 10-year interdisciplinary study of older people confirmed what Masters and Johnson found, that is, that older people remain interested in sexual activities. However, similar to Kinsey they found that older men were more involved in sexual activity than women. In fact, an interesting finding of the study showed that 13 to 15% of their sample showed an increase in sexual activity and interest with advancing age. Impaired sexual functioning was related to the male's health, cognition, and social situation.

Starr (1981) and Brecher (1984) are two very recent studies related to geriatric sexuality. They found that men are now more sexually active than in Kinsey's time. However, both studies found that there is declining sexual activity with age.

In summation, the three factors that seem to predict sexual activity for the older male and female are prior interest, physical health, and an available partner. However, a major limitation of these studies is that they focused on genital sex rather than relationships and sexual satisfaction via other modes of expression.

PHYSICAL CHANGES

What happens as we physically age? The neurophysiology of both males and females is the result of an interplay between the nervous system, the vascular system, and the endocrine system. These three systems also interact with both the interpsychic and social environment of the patient. Although studies show that there are consistent physiological changes in the sexual response cycle with aging, these changes do not occur with all patients and there are varying degrees of change between individuals. These changes do not typically cause the cessation of sexual activity for most individuals.

The Older Woman and Sexuality

By the time older women have reached 65, many have been experiencing the long-term effects of menopause. As discussed in the prior chapter, menopause has many significant implications for sexuality. These include changes in the sexual response cycle, body image alterations, and changes in the genito-urinary system that may foster more infections and pain with intercourse.

Because of the lack of estrogen and the resulting loss of lubrication during the sexual excitement and orgasm phase, sexual problems may occur. This depletion may cause dyspareunia or painful intercourse. Estrogen depletion can also cause vaginitis.

One of the most effective nursing interventions for the relief of dyspareunia is to discuss with the woman the use of lubricants. There are several over-the-counter interventions on the market. These are water-soluble lubricants which can be used prior to intercourse or even when the woman feels uncomfortably dry. They are usually packaged to look like a tampon and are easy and safe to insert. Vaseline should not be used in the vaginal canal because it is not water soluble and therefore can precipitate infections.

Other changes in the reproductive tract influence changes in the orgasmic contractions of the uterus that occur during the orgasmic phase of the sexual response cycle. In the young woman, the uterus tents (rises) and contracts during orgasm. This is usually perceived as a pleasurable and intense experience. With aging these contractions can become very painful and may cause sexual discomfort. Eventually a sexual dysfunction may occur if the woman becomes fearful and avoids sex because it is perceived as painful.

Another problem related to aging is dysuria, which is caused by irritation of the urethra, the urinary bladder opening. Urinary dribbling caused by hypotonia may also occur and may ultimately lead to frequent urinary infections and incontinence. The fear of incontinence and also the concurrent smell related to incontinence can also inhibit sexual desire for both partners.

Informing the female patient to void before intercourse is helpful in preventing urinary infections. Teaching women "tightening" exercises for the perineum such as the Kegel exercise may help tighten the vaginal canal and help make intercourse more pleasurable.

There are several other nursing implications related to women, aging and sexuality. The adage "use it or lose it" applies to women as well as to men. Regular sexual activity that includes intercourse at least once or twice a week is important. A longer period of time for foreplay and other pregenital sexual activities will also enhance sexual enjoyment. Sexual activity seems to delay and/or modify the changes of menopause in a positive way. (See Table 7-1.) Post menopausal women that are sexually active have less shrinkage of the vagina and higher levels of androgens and pituitary gonadatropins (LH and FSH) than sexually inactive women.

Table 7—1
Nursing Interventions to Enhance Female Sexuality

The following suggestions can be helpful guidelines for your female patients toward maintaining sexual expression.

1. Consider sexuality to be as important to the relationship as sexual intercourse.

2. Recognize the mind-body connection.

3. Communicate to your partner your sexual preferences and desires.

4. Lead a "balanced" life.

5. Maintain good nutrition.

6. Nurture your relationship.

7. Use all five senses to create desire.

8. Have adequate information related to the normal physiological changes that occur during the aging process.

9. Use lubricants or estrogen replacement therapy (if indicated).

10. Practice peritoneum-tightening exercises.

11. Have more time for foreplay and pregenital activity so that adequate lubrication can occur.

12. Empty your bladder before intercourse.

13. Engage in regular sexual activity.

The Older Man and Sexuality

The older male also experiences physical changes as a result of the aging process, many of which are related to changes in the sexual response cycle. Older men seem to have a less intense physiological response during the excitement phase of the sexual response cycle. This means that it takes longer for an erection to occur.

It is very important to realize that few older men can "will" an erection. During adolescence and young adulthood, erections occur quickly and fully with minimal thought and visual and sensual stimulation. The older male and his partner must realize that it takes more time and more mutual stimulation to have and to maintain an erection. If the older male does not realize this crucial fact and if his spouse or partner is uninterested in having sexual intercourse or is in a hurry "to get it over with," the proper mind-body response cycle will not occur and the male will not attain an erection.

As a result of this experience, the elderly male may consider himself a failure and avoid trying to have sex altogether. Or, he may desperately attempt to have sexual intercourse with a girlfriend, or even in extreme cases a prostitute. This usually is a failure as well because the prostitute is "uncaring" and even in more of a hurry than his spouse. Or he may attempt to have "an affair" with a mutual friend, neighbor, or coworker. This also usually ends in failure because guilt and performance anxiety overwhelm him with stress, thus preventing an erection from occurring. What the older male really needs is a loving, understanding, willing spouse or partner.

Normally during sleep, men experience penile tumescence (rigidity). This occurs during the rapid eye movement (REM) period of sleep. The total amount of REM-related nocturnal penile temescence declines throughout the life cycle. The erection that was always present in the morning may no longer occur. For many men and women this is symbolic of a great decline in sexual health. Men may also be slower to experience orgasms as they age, and when they do have an orgasm it may feel less intense. Men over the age of 60 may also have a weaker ejaculatory experience. The force and volume of seminal fluid may become reduced, with less of a need to ejaculate with every sexual encounter. Another physical change which also involves the sexual response cycle involves the refractory period, the period of time that typically occurs after orgasm. In the young man, this period can be very short and erection can occur almost immediately again. In the older adult, the refractory phase becomes greatly prolonged. The implication of this change is that if erection is lost during the excitement phase, it may takes many hours before the man can have another erection.

Older men also experience some mild hormonal changes. As they age, there appears to be less available testosterone. However, only a small amount of men over the age of 50 have been found to have abnormal hormone levels that would impair sexual functioning.

Both men and women also begin to experience chronic diseases as they age. Many of these diseases, such as hypertension, diabetes, prostate enlargement in the male, and heart disease, can negatively affect sexual expression. Both the physical process and the treatment for chronic disease can also influence the sexual response cycle.

Thus men, like women, need information regarding what normal sexual aging encompasses. Whenever possible it is important to include your patient's partner in sexual health teaching and counseling.

For example, it is important to encourage older men to take "advantage" of an erection. It is also important to teach the couple to become aware of the time of day that they feel is least stressful and when they are feeling the most alert. Since more penile stimulation is frequently necessary to achieve an erection, it is important that the patient be aware of this fact. This knowledge may make him feel more comfortable in asking for more direct stimulation. Adding oral or mechanical devices such as vibrators to sexual foreplay can also be helpful. Having the partner be more aware of these changes will help her feel less responsible.

Here also the adage "use it or lose it" is appropriate. When possible, sexual activity should occur at least once a week. It is also important to stress to the elderly male that alcohol should be avoided prior to inter-course because although it may increase desire it may also prevent erection.

Because the sexual changes in the male are so much more obvious than in the female, males cannot "fake" sexual arousal. Unfortunately, this is sometimes interpreted by the sexual partner to mean that the male is no longer interested in sex or that he may even be having an affair. Thus, it is crucial to encourage open, honest conversation. Unfortunately, for many of our older patients this conversation may be very embarrassing. Many in this group are not comfortable talking about their sexual needs. We need to be sensitive to this discomfort and respect the boundaries that they set. Sometimes, because of the anxiety level, it is helpful to give this information in a few sessions rather than one very intensive session.

For a summary of interventions for men, see Table 7-2. Table 7-3 presents an overview of how aging affects both men and women.

Table 7—2
Nursing Interventions to Enhance Male Sexuality

1. Consider sexuality to be as important to a relationship as is sexual intercourse.

2. Recognize the mind-body connection.

3. Maintain good nutrition.

4. Nurture your relationship.

5. Have accurate information.

6. Engage in regular sexual activity: at least once or twice a week.

7. Take "advantage" of an erection.

8. Have intercourse when the highest energy level is present.

9. Avoid alcohol.

10. Use more direct penile stimulation.

11. Be aware of medication's effect on sexuality.

12. Use all five senses to create desire.

Table 7–3
The Effect of Aging on the Sexual Response Cycle

Males	Females
Desire	
May be diminished as a result of drugs, chronic disease, loss of partner or lack of partner, depression, fatigue, and body image changes of self and/or partner.	

Males	Females
Excitement	
Sex flush does not always occur	There is less vaginal lubrication
Penile erection may be less firm	More time is needed for adequate lubrication.
More direct stimulation of the penis is needed to obtain a full erection.	Vasocongestion of the labia minora decreases
	Vaginal ballooning is delayed.
	Vasocongestion of the breasts is diminished.
	Less muscle tension.

Males	Females
Plateau	
Testicular elevation is reduced.	The vaginal barrel does not widen or elongate.
Scrotal wall vasocongestionis reduced.	Elevation of labia majora is decreased.
	There is no sex flush.
	There is less muscle tension.

Table 7–3 (continued)
The Effect of Aging on the Sexual Response Cycle

Orgasm

Males	Females
Ejaculatory strength is reduced.	Vasocongestion is decreased.
Penile contractions are fewer.	Fewer vaginal contractions occur.
There is diminished sensation of ejaculatory inevitability.	Uterine contractions may be painful or feel more intense.
Erection is lost more quickly.	Vaginal balloon shrinks rapidly.
	Increased urinary frequency.
	Dysuria increases.

Refractory

Refractory period is prolonged.	There is no refractory period in women.

Adapted from Masters, W.M. & Johnson, V.E. *Human Sexual Response.* Boston: Little, Brown & Co. 1966.

CONCLUSION

Aging does not necessitate the end of a sexual life, but it may pose a critical challenge to sexuality because of certain psychosocial and biological changes. Nurses and other health care professionals should have the professional knowledge to help minimize these effects. There are now many kinds of self-help books that are available, and using books may be less anxiety provoking and therefore more useful than direct counseling. Another interesting idea for nursing would be to create sex education programs for older patients in which they could learn and process the information needed to enhance their sexuality.

However, the most crucial concern of nurses should be to help patients feel entitled to, and experience their sexuality in a positive and pleasurable manner. Finally, we need to be respectful of the needs of our elderly patients and not negate their rights to sexual expression.

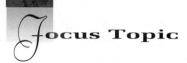

Focus Topic

Sex and the Older Marriage

There are very few broad generalizations that can be made regarding the nature of sex and the older marriage. In fact, there is a large amount of disagreement as to whether marriages that have been together for 30 or more years actually increase or decrease in marital or sexual satisfaction. What is known about the older marriage is that the older couple typically experiences more losses due to aging, chronic illness, and all of the other life situations that go along with advancing age.

Couples, at this juncture of time, are also more likely to have fairly definite ways of relating to one another. In other words, the angry, conflictual marriage is less likely to resolve this pattern of interaction, and the open and honest relationship is less likely to become conflictual. Major relational changes do not occur at this late age.

Divorce is also much more unlikely at this point in life, perhaps because older people are typically coping with many involuntary losses and may be hesitant to risk a life change that may create other losses in their lives. Adult children are frequently against divorce in their aging parents and will frequently be very forceful toward "not allowing" their parents to divorce.

All of these life stressors can create increased anger in couples, especially if they have not learned how to communicate in a positive way. As in younger couples, sex is frequently the first casualty in a marital war. Unfortunately, some research is finding that for the older couple it is more difficult to resume sex once it has been given up for a period of time. Finally, health problems may cause role reversals in couple dynamics and frequently wives will take on the role of mother, or husbands the role of father.

There are also positive factors in an older marriage. These include the capacity for a greater acceptance of each other and a increased willingness to compromise. The family history that the partners have created together also helps create generativity and gives meaning to their lives.

Sex is not typically as necessary for marital expression or satisfaction as in earlier years. Significantly, in the older couple sex as a learned pattern of pleasure becomes more crucial than direct genital arousal.

There is also a mind-body connection that seems to become more important as we age. If the couple has had a past history of pleasure with their sexuality, they will be more likely to continue this behavior as they age. Middle age seems to be the important determinant as to whether a couple will continue with their sexual intimacy.

Other factors which may hinder sexual expression include lack of knowledge regarding aging and sexuality and ignorance or "buying in" to ageist beliefs and physical illness. If the couple believes that "sex is dirty for older people," this obviously will greatly hinder their sexual expression. Lack of good communication skills can also be a deterrent if the couple cannot communicate their changing sexual needs with one another.

However, couples who have had a history of prior good sex lives may be open and willing to come to a health professional for help regarding their sexual health as they age.

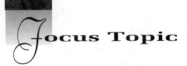

Focus Topic

An Overview of Aging

Object-relations: This period will bring an incorporation of one's self concept in terms of positive acceptance.

Erikson: This is the Stage of Integrity vs. Despair. It is during this stage where many adults begin to initiate a life review. In this review they many begin to work through issues related to what they have achieved in terms of personal and professional satisfaction; what they have contributed and where they have failed. If they feel satisfied in the meaning of their lives they will have achieved the task of this stage.

Family life cycle: Launching children and moving on; the family in later life.

Tasks of this stage include: working through issues of mortality; coming to spiritual peace; viewing death in peace rather than in fear; accepting one's limitations; not disengaging or separating from the world; coping with an aging body; letting go of children; coping with multiple losses; grandparenting; creating a life after retirement.

Sexuality: Sex life can continue; adjusting to an older body and changing body image; adjusting and finding new ways to express sexuality if it has been challenged by disease; finding oneself in new intimate relationships; adjusting to new relationships such as widowhood, etc.

Stressors related to illness: Coping with multiple losses; accepting the loss of power and health; changing one's diet and activity level; adjusting to a new life style; fiances; inability to possibly travel; coping with body image changes; living within an aegist population; possibly being placed within a nursing home.

Part III

Medical Issues and Sexuality

Mrs. G had just been discharged from the hospital. This was her first night at home. Just 10 days ago she had suffered a myocardial infarction. She was tired and still feeling scared about the experience. That night, when her husband reached out to hold her, she trembled and withdrew. After all, she thought, what if having sex would cause her to have another heart attack? She moved further away. Her husband stayed awake through the night wondering why she was angry with him.

Mr. G had diabetes since he was 12 years old. Now, after his divorce at the age of 40, he was beginning to date again. He really enjoyed being with this woman he had just met but there was so much he hadn't shared with her about his sexuality. How could he explain to his new girlfriend that sometimes he could not have an erection? How could he explain the term *retrograde ejaculation*? He hadn't heard about that condition until it had happened to him. Would she understand? What if she wanted to have children? Would she think that he was a freak?

Mrs. W was 65. She had just had a hysterectomy and had her uterus and ovaries removed. She couldn't stop feeling a tremendous sadness. She told herself that she was acting silly. After all, she had two beautiful children and six grandchildren. Yet it was that uterus that had cradled her children through nine months of pregnancy.

This part of the book will present information related to medical illness and its impact upon sexual functioning. Nurses need to be aware of the unique problems and challenges that chronically ill patients may have expressing their sexuality, since each disease process may also have specific mechanisms that may affect sexual functioning. As professional nurses we need to be informed of these physiological and psychological influences and changes so that our patients will have the information they need to cope and adapt to various illnesses.

Unlike Part II, this section of the book is not based on a life cycle perspective. Since illness does not respect age barriers, it frequently affects the young as well as the very old. However, it may be helpful to refer to the developmental issues previously discussed.

Chapter 8

Challenges to Sexuality

MYTHS ABOUT SEXUALITY AND ILLNESS

There are many common myths or belief systems regarding sexual functioning and illness. We need to be aware of their presence when working with the patient who is ill because these myths frequently influence a patient's sexual expression and level of comfort with sex. They include the following beliefs:

Sex is only for the young and able-bodied.

Sex means only intercourse.

The goal of sexual activity is orgasm.

Sexual activity must be natural and spontaneous.

Masturbation is harmful.

We need to be aware of our own personal values as well as any underlying prejudices we may consciously or unconsciously harbor regarding sexual expression because our personal attitudes frequently influence the care that we give our patients.

Medical illness frequently challenges our moral, ethical, and cultural belief systems. For example, if orgasm is the perceived goal of sexuality and patients are unable to have an orgasm, we may need to shift their focus from this goal to some alternative behaviors that may give pleasure, such as touching, hugging, or kissing. However, if we are not comfortable with our own sexuality or believe any of the above myths, we may be ineffective and even destructive in our interventions.

For example, a nurse who believes that procreation or childbearing is the only proper basis for sexual activity may communicate these feelings to the patient. Since many patients become infertile as a result of a disease process or treatment, such an attitude can be harmful. Finally, if nurses believe that sex is only for those patients under the age of 40, they need to be aware of how ageism may affect their attitudes and the information that they share with older patients.

The rest of this chapter reviews some of the emotional and physical challenges that may occur as the result of illness and that frequently affect sexual functioning. The effect of these changes can be short-term or longer-termed, catastrophic or manageable. Changes may have minimal effect on sexual functioning or make the person feel asexual. However, illness will typically affect sexuality to some degree. For a model as an example of some of the different variables that can be involved, see Figure 8-1. When assessing a patient, this model can be a helpful reminder toward evaluating the patient in a more comprehensive manner.

FIGURE 8—1
The Impact of an Illness on Sexuality: A Woman with a Hysterectomy and Lack of Desire

TIME FACTOR

History	Patients Age	Duration of Symptoms
Since 1991	44	1992

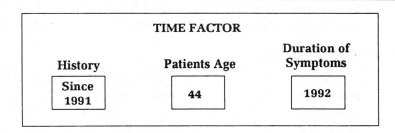

MORAL
- Roman Catholic
- Sex For Procreation

PSYCHOLOGICAL
- Sex Role Conflict
- Self Esteem
- Poor Body Image
- Anger
- Depression

BIOLOGICAL
- Weight Gain
- Hot Flashes
- Dysparunia
- Lubrication

SOCIAL
- 4 Children All Teenagers
- Marital Relationship Poor
- Aging Parents
- Good Economic Status
- Homemaker
- Northern European

EMOTIONAL REACTIONS TO ILLNESS

There are many factors that influence patients' reactions to an illness. Their previous coping style is very likely to determine to some degree how they will cope with their new demands. Other factors include the quality and commitment of the important relationships in their life, their gender, their ethnicity, and their religion. Sociocultural and economic class will also influence how patients react. Nurses should consider all these factors when developing a nursing care plan for patients and their families.

The following emotions are frequently experienced during an illness. These emotional responses often have a negative effect on not only sexual expression but also on quality of life and self-esteem.

Anger

"Why me?" The amount of anger expressed or experienced is usually related to several factors. These may include age and marital status, the effect that the disease will have on patients' lives (medically and sexually), and the effect it will have upon their families (financially and socially).

For example, a women who is 60 years old and experiences a hysterectomy usually feels less anger over the loss of her uterus than a younger woman who has not had any children. A 15-year-old juvenile-onset, insulin-dependent diabetic may be more angry about "life" than a 75-year-old woman who develops adult-onset, non-insulin-dependent diabetes during older age.

Another very important point to consider, as noted by the author after years of counseling patients, is that in all relationships where strong angry feelings are experienced, anger is a third person in the couple's bed. Frequently the spouse is the target of a patient's anger. A satisfying relationship is therefore almost impossible to achieve until the issues that cause or aggravate the anger are resolved. This may be especially true when lifestyle behaviors have contributed to causing the illness.

For example, anger is frequently experienced by the spouse of an alcoholic who now has cirrhosis, or the spouse of a patient who has smoked and now has lung cancer. Anger can be even more destructive when a disease is sexually transmitted. This is especially relevant in this era of AIDS.

Confusion

Confusion is an emotion that is frequently felt when there are many "unknowns" regarding prognosis. Patients may have many questions regarding the implications of the disease process on their quality of life, including their sexuality. A common example of this situation is the young man with diabetes, who may or may not have experienced the side-effect of neuropathy, which affects erection and ejaculation.

Denial

Denial is an inevitable reaction for many patients, especially when they suddenly become ill. "It can't be me. . . it must be a mistake." This can have a negative effect on patients' ability to cope with the illness. They may suddenly exhibit bizarre or inappropriate behavior such as lavish spending sprees, avoid traditional medical care in favor of faith healers or mystics, or even try to act 20 years younger both physically and sexually to prove that they are not ill at all.

Fear

Fear is a important emotion to consider when addressing the needs of all patients. They may be worried that they will become increasingly dependent on others because of their perceived impending or progressive disability. They may also fear the pain of progressive disease and/or treatment. For example, the cancer patient who needs to have chemotherapy or radiation may be mentally paralyzed with the fear of the treatment and the potential side-effects of therapy.

People who are fearful react in different ways in terms of sexual expression. Some patients seek increased sexual intimacy. This reaction may be seen as a reenactment of when they were children and felt safe in their mother's arms. Other patients may react totally differently and distance themselves from their loved ones and not want to be touched nor held.

Sex is sometimes viewed as a life-sustaining statement: It is frequently associated or related to being healthy and therefore connected to life. For some patients, therefore; the expression of sexuality may be interpreted as an affirmation that they are not gravely sick. Patients who are very fearful of dying may embrace this belief system as a means of coping with their fear.

Shame

Shame is a very negative and destructive emotion that can be frequently experienced throughout the life cycle. For example, the young child may experience shame as a result of invasive procedures in the hospital. This childhood sense of shame can even affect sexual expression in later adult life in terms of sexual satisfaction and enjoyment. The adult who is feeling embarrassed may continue or begin to avoid intimacy as an adult.

The older adult can also experience shame as a result of an illness. The obvious medical or surgical loss of a major organ (bladder—ureterostomy; bowel—colostomy or ileostomy; sexual organs— testicular implants) with a silicone implant, plastic bag, or rubber ball such as penis—balloon pump implant can have a major negative effect upon sexual expression, sense of self-esteem, and entitlement to sexual satisfaction.

Guilt

Many patients believe that they are responsible for their disease. These patients may include obese men and women, heavy smokers, and AIDS victims who failed to use safer sex practices. They may feel not only guilt related to becoming a "burden" to their families but also shame if they develop an illness that they believe was caused by their behavior. These negative self-concepts may have a destructive influence on sexual activity and relationships because they cause feelings of denial, withdrawal, self-pity, and depression.

Loss of control

Most people need a sense of control in their lives, and patients also need to control their environment. Illness can challenge patients' sense of their sex role and self-concept. Being or becoming dependent on others and possibly losing an influential role in the family or at work can influence relationships and self-esteem. Being considered the "sick" person is frequently a very destructive concept that precipitates a sense of multiple losses. These losses can trigger both anxiety and hopelessness.

Depression

Chronically ill patients are frequently depressed. Although depression is really a symptom complex, its most consistent feature is hopelessness. The prevalence of depression within a hospital setting ranges from 13% to more than 70%. This estimate varies because the symptoms of depression are often the same as those of physical illness. Frequently, therefore, a careful history needs to be taken to diagnose depression.

Depression or sad affect is frequently seen in patients with chronic or life-threatening disease. These depressions are frequently called secondary or "reactive" depressions because the etiology of the disease is related to an adverse life experience. Depression can lead to a lower sense of sexual desire because depressed patients frequently disengage themselves from the world and the people around them.

Depression is frequently experienced as the result of loss. The more "losses" that patients experience as a result of illness, the more likely it is that they will become depressed and withdrawn.

There are many symptoms of depression. However, the most common symptom is sad affect related to loss of pleasure in everyday life activities. Other symptoms include sleep disorders (too much sleep, too little sleep, early morning awakening, and difficulty in falling asleep), eating disorders (anorexia or overeating), anxiety, changes in cognitive functioning, physical disorders (headache, stomachache, and back pain), and lack of desire to relate to family or friends.

Depression frequently needs to be treated. This may be done through counseling, support groups, and/or psychotrophic medications. Although there has been debate over the success of using medication with reactive depression, it has been found to be frequently beneficial. It is the author's opinion that any patient who is placed on medication for depression also needs counseling to help create insight, facilitate grieving if necessary, maintain self-esteem in the face of multiple losses related to physical illness, and remain in "touch" with their feelings.

THE ROLE OF THE FAMILY

Some of the most important variables that can affect sexual functioning are the history, belief system, cultural attitudes, and behaviors of the patient's family. For example, if the family medical genogram (history) has several male members who died suddenly from heart disease while having sex, or female members who had a mastectomy as a result of breast cancer, when patients are diagnosed with one of these illnesses their reaction and expectations may be affected by what know happened to these other family members. If family experiences have been negative, they may expect to have the same experience.

Families also have cultural and religious attitudes regarding sexual expression. These attitudes may be enabling or fatalistic. If the family is not supportive in helping patients or couples seek out sexual counseling, they may not do so, and therefore they may not take advantage of all of the medical and social interventions available to enhance their sexuality.

Since families are closed systems (what happens to one member will influence other members), the advent of a acute or chronic disease may affect the sexuality of other members of the family. For example:

> June is 39 and Rick is 42. They have three children, ages 18, 14, and 12. One year ago, the youngest daughter, Emily, had been diagnosed with cancer. Since Emily's diagnosis then the whole family felt depressed. As a result of that depression, June gained 30 pounds and Rick gained 20 pounds. The oldest daughter, Terry, stopped dating because she wanted to be with her sister. The middle daughter, Carole, seems to be okay but has many stomachaches. June and Rick are too tired to have sex; it just isn't a priority. In fact, they haven't been sexual in 4 months.

Other ongoing stressors can also affect how the family copes with sexuality. If the family is already stressed to the maximum, sex may be the last priority for the couple. For example, it may feel very unimportant in the family with a great amount of alcoholism or physical or sexual abuse. Family members who are coping with multiple stressors and illnesses at the same time frequently have low sexual desire.

It is useful to remember, in this connection, that even normal developmental events can cause stress in a family. These stressors may include "happy" events such as weddings and the birth of children or grandchildren.

Whenever possible, it is very helpful for the nurse to talk to all members of the family. Even watching a family interact or sitting with the family for a short period of time can give you invaluable information regarding how the illness may be affecting not only the patient but also other members of the family.

BODY IMAGE CHANGES

Threats to body image can be one of the most destructive influences on positive self-concept and sexual expression. There are several variables that can affect self-concept. Changes in body image can be real, perceived, or even fantasized. Some of the guidelines to consider when assessing for threats to body image and their impact upon the patient include the following:

1. Are the changes observable? A woman who has had a mastectomy is frequently perceived as being traumatized because the surgery causes a very observable change in her body (the loss of a breast) as well as loss of a body part that has great symbolic meaning in our culture. Because her loss is frequently acknowledged by the health professional and her family she will usually be given a greater opportunity to discuss her feelings.

2. Are the changes to the body functional? The removal of a gall bladder may cause a negative body image change because there is an obvious scar. However, this surgery is usually far less traumatic to the patient than the removal of a uterus in a 20-year-old woman or the loss of kidney function in any age group. Nonfunctional body image changes do not typically affect the quality of life.

3. Is the loss symbolic? An example of a symbolic body image loss is the 60-year-old wife who has had a hysterectomy or the 70-year-old man who has had a bilateral orchiectomy due to prostate cancer. Although she can no longer have children, due to menopause, she may still feel depressed. Although his sperm count declined many years ago, he may also become very depressed. If fertility, motherhood, and fatherhood had been an important part of their self-concept, they will experience these surgeries as an assault on their body image.

4. Is the change temporary? Being incapacitated in a leg cast for 6 weeks is usually less traumatic than developing a buffalo hump from osteoporosis. The adolescent who has had a colostomy as a result of ulcerative colitis may be very worried about his future dating and sexual performance. However, even some temporary changes can be very traumatic. Hair loss due to chemotherapy is usually a significant threat to body image. Weight gain related to chemotherapy medication may also be only temporary but may cause serious body image distortion.

5. Is the loss permanent? Losing a leg because of cardiovascular disease, a kidney because of renal disease, or a bladder because of bladder cancer will challenge not only patients' sense of positive body image but also the coping abilities of themselves and their family. Adjustment is usually more difficult with permanent losses.

6. Is the illness socially acceptable? Gall bladder disease, diabetes, and hypertension are considered socially acceptable diseases; depression, epilepsy, ulcerative colitis, herpes, and AIDS are not. A diagnosis of these latter diseases may therefore elicit a negative societal reaction. Patients and their families may feel disapproval and embarrassment from their friends and even the nursing staff. The etiology of the disease also may affect not only the patients' and their families' self-concept but also the attitudes of professionals who care for them. For example, attitudes toward patients who have acquired AIDS through a blood transfusion will differ from attitudes toward those who have acquired AIDS through the use of contaminated needles.

7. Is the patient feeling dehumanized as a result of the hospital or medical experience? Being the "breast cancer" in room 447 can challenge a woman's sense of femininity and intimacy. The lack of privacy for the hospitalized patient can also hinder intimacy even in terms of hugging or being held. Sharing a room with another person also alters the ability of a couple to have a private conversation and to address issues of intimacy and feeling with one another.

8. What life cycle body images are occurring? Changes related to aging can be negative threats to body image. As discussed, we are an ageist culture, and we are not comfortable with the normal changes of aging. Compounding these threats, the concurrent body image changes related to a disease process may make the older patient feel extremely vulnerable.

In conclusion, both chronic and acute illness can trigger an array of feelings, including depression, anxiety, denial, sadness, anger, guilt, and shame. They can also cause numerous threats to body image. The consequences of these psychological reactions are numerous. They frequently affect sexuality and patients' sense of themselves as positive sexual beings.

PHYSICAL SIDE-EFFECTS OF ILLNESS

There are several physical side-effects of illness that can influence the sexuality of the patient and the couple.

Pain is present in most illnesses. For example, the pain of a swollen knee due to arthritis may be very incapacitating and may also hinder sexual desire and performance. Pain may also be caused by medical testing. An example of a painful procedure during the diagnosis process is a bone marrow test, which is used to confirm the diagnosis of Hodgkin's disease and leukemia. Pain is a frequent factor in causing sexual dysfunctions and may be a catalyst for lack of desire and intimacy.

Fatigue, also found in a wide range of illnesses, can cause a marked decrease in the level of sexual functioning. This can also be true for the partner who is the patient's caregiver if they are also not getting enough rest or sleep.

The more chronic the disease process, the more likely it is that there will be stress, anxiety, and tension between partners. Chronicity will also influence a patient's sense of privacy, since many of the family members may become involved with the care or caregiving of the patient and the couple. As a result, patients may lose their sense of adulthood and feel more childlike and less sexual.

Implications for Nursing

The above discussion highlights some of the key issues related to illness and sexual functioning. It is crucial that nurses assess those issues that they believe may be affecting patients and be knowledgeable about the kinds of changes that patients can make.

For example, if a patient states that she is experiencing pain with intercourse because of a mastectomy scar, the nurse can recommend a sexual position in which the partner is not putting any pressure on this incision. Another example of a positive nursing intervention is to suggest that the patient who is incontinent void before intercourse. A third intervention could be to suggest making love in the morning when the patient with a heart condition may feel less fatigued. Remember, many patients are afraid or ashamed to ask questions. Positive interventions include both the physical and emotional concerns of patients and their significant others.

By giving patients clear, factual information, we are giving them permission to ask questions regarding their sexuality. Nurses need to ascertain not only what accurate information patients have, but also what myths and beliefs are part of their and their families' belief system. Identifying negative influences helps patients resolve these issues. Discussion also serves as modeling behavior for family members who may have discomfort in addressing very sensitive issues.

Patients who have had a positive sexual history prior to an illness are frequently well motivated and willing to make changes in their behavior so that they can maintain a level of sexual functioning. It is important to encourage patients to resume sexual activity as soon as possible after convalescence so that they can maintain sexual functioning and intimacy. Research has documented that the longer a couple delays resuming intimacy, the more difficult it becomes to be sexual again. For the older couple, the old adage "use it or lose it" is especially applicable.

Sex and the Patient with Cardiovascular Disease

Mr. A had not been feeling well for the past 6 months. So he wasn't too shocked when the nurse told him that his blood pressure was 160/100. However, when he started to describe all of the physical changes that he had been feeling, he realized that he had also been having problems getting an erection. He wondered if there was any connection between all of these new medical problems.

It has been estimated that over 63 million Americans have one or more types of heart or blood vessel disease. One in four adults has hypertension, and 2 million people have rheumatic heart disease. Heart disease is of epidemic proportions in the United States.

Physical limitations related to poor circulation, medication side-effects and poor physical stamina influence sexual functioning for the cardiovascular patient. However, the fear of having another heart attack while having sex is typically what causes most people to abstain from sex.

MYOCARDIAL INFARCTION

Unfortunately, after a myocardial infarction many patients do not resume sex because they do not get adequate information regarding **when** and **how** they can engage in sexual intercourse. Many believe that sex may precipitate symptoms, cause another myocardial infarction, or cause sudden death. To further compound the problem, many patients are uncomfortable asking health professionals about sexual concerns. And typically when a "conspiracy of silence" occurs in the sexual arena, sexual activity stops.

Physiological Responses

According to the studies of Masters and Johnson (1966), certain physiological changes occur during the sexual response cycle. In the arousal period there is a skin flush, an increased sense of warmth, increased respiration, increased heart rate, and elevated blood pressure. This increased rate of physiological function continues until orgasm. At that time the maximum respiratory rate goes from 16 to 60 respirations per minute, the heart rate goes from 70 to 170 beats per minute, and the blood pressure goes from 120/80 to peak levels of 220/110. However, within seconds after orgasm the physiological changes that have occurred begin to normalize.

It is important to "qualify" these physiological findings with the fact that the physical changes just described were monitored in a hospital research laboratory setting. Other studies have been done under less artificial settings that have showed lower levels of physiological change.

What has been ascertained from the data is that for the average, middle-aged long-married man or woman with cardiovascular disease there is low physiological cost to sexual intercourse. It has also been concluded that climbing two flights of stairs following a 10-minute brisk walk is one guideline of determining a patient's readiness for sexual activity. Another medical finding that help create less stress for the male with a myocardial infarction is the information that the "upper" position for the woman during sex demands less energy for the male.

A definite risk factor with angina or myocardial infarction, however, is having sex with an extramarital partner or in an unfamiliar setting: the "motel coronary." The stress, guilt, time pressure and anxiety of a one night stand causes a marked outpouring or adrenaline from the adrenal gland. Adrenaline then stimulates the entire nervous system, causing an increased heart rate, elevated blood pressure with possible secondary palpitations, arrythmias, coronary artery spasm, and even sudden death. However, even for couples in long term relationships, the fear of a "coital coronary" still remains and needs to be discussed.

Psychological Responses

Research has documented many different emotional responses of both patients and their partners after a myocardial infarction. The most common responses are anxiety, depression, and fear. Depression is often experienced as patients begin to comprehend the potential for multiple losses in their lives.

Although this is a less common reaction, some patients deny their illness and then become angry, guilty, and/or sexually aggressive. Anger and resentment are unfortunate, but common reactions to a myocardial infarction. When they are identified in a patient, it is important that these emotions are addressed and not ignored.

Patients as well as their partners are confronted with emotional issues related to mortality, dependency, loss, and changing roles. A common occurrence for men who have experienced a myocardial infarction is that their wives become overprotective and take on the role of "mother." Obviously this role is not conducive to sexual intimacy or sexual desire. This behavior needs to be discussed because of its potential for creating unhealthy relationship dynamics.

Implications for Nursing

The overall goal for the nurse is to help patients and their families develop good coping skills so that they can adjust to the illness in a more positive way.

Information regarding sexual activity should begin early in the hospitalization period. There are several reasons for early intervention, the most important being to give patients a sense of hope in the future. Giving patients and their significant others time to process anxiety-producing information in an accurate manner and dispelling the myths that they may have heard from friends or patients are other important reasons for early intervention.

A frequently overlooked behavior that can be helpful for the cardiac patient is masturbation. Until recently this has been a taboo topic. Initially, after a myocardial infarction, there may be very little sexual interest. However, when patients begin to ambulate again and feel that they will "survive," sexual interest may re-develop. This may be very reassuring and give them the sense that once again they are connected to life.

Interviews with patients who have had cardiac problems indicate that it is not uncommon for them to masturbate while they are still in the hospital. Since this can be interpreted by patients as a continuation of their sex life, introducing the therapeutic use of masturbation as a method of reentering sexual activity may be beneficial. Studies related to the physiological changes that occur during masturbation have shown that the heart rate typically does not go above 130 beats per minute. Therefore, when the physician feels that the patient can meet this physiological challenge he can recommend masturbation to the patient. This permission giving can be very important for the patient who needs to connect with his sexuality.

Giving accurate information regarding medications is another important nursing function. It is important to preface this section with the comment that many of the medications can actually improve sexual functioning by increasing exercise tolerance and cardiac reserve. However, we live in a "drug-phobic society." It is commonly misperceived, especially by the elderly, that all medications affect sexuality in a negative way. This needs to be discussed because many patients do not comply with their medications out of fear and ignorance. They believe that if they take their medicine they will never be sexual again.

The following antihypertensive medications have been known to affect sexual functioning. This is not a totally inclusive list. These sympatholytic agents act directly on either the central nervous system or the autonomic nervous system (*sympatholytic* means "to cut the sympathetic nerve" reflex stimuli). These medications fall into five categories:

1. Central-acting agents
   a. Methyldopa (Aldomet)
   b. Clonidine hydrochloride (Catapres)
   c. Reserpine

2. Beta-adrenergic blocking agents
   a. Propranolol hydrochloride (Inderal)
   b. Metoprolol tartrate (Lopressor)
   c. Atenolol (Tenormin)

3. Alpha-adrenergic blocking agents
   a. Prazosin hydrochloride (Minipress)

4. Mixed alpha- and beta-adrenergic blocking agents
   a. Labetalol hydrochloride (Normodyne/Trandate)

5. Peripherally acting sympatholytic agents
   a. Guanethidine sulfate (Ismelin)

(This is not a totally inclusive list.)

These drugs in susceptible patients can cause various degrees of inhibited desire, erectile dysfunction, and ejaculatory failure. Other classes of hypertensive drugs, such as diuretics, angiotension converting enzyme (ACE) inhibitors, calcium channel blockers, may occasionally cause sexual dysfunction in various degrees. Often, however, the effects of these medications are dose related.

It is important for patients to understand that in the majority of cases, when drugs are taken correctly, they will increase exercise reserve and control angina. This will then result in enhanced sexual functioning. Therefore, proper medication can actually benefit the patients' sexuality in a positive way.

Improved exercise tolerance and a life-style that balances work with leisure time are also important. Not smoking and drinking less alcohol are important variables for patients to consider. All of these lifestyle changes need to be discussed by nurses if we are to participate in pre vention-focused care.

HYPERTENSION

Hypertension, the "silent killer," affects approximately 55 million adults in the United States. However, for many of these people it is undetected and does not send them to the hospital until they develop severe symptoms such as angina, myocardial infarction, renal failure, and stroke.

Sexual Counseling

There are two important considerations for nurses to remember regarding sexual counseling and the hypertensive patient. The first is that blood pressure is indeed the "silent killer;" therefore, it is important to emphasize compliance in taking medications so that the patient's blood pressure is under control at all times. This should definitely help extend the patient's life expectancy.

Patients may also need to be counseled regarding life-style and habit changes. Concerns related to weight control and cigarette smoking may need to be discussed. Suggestions for support groups, weight loss programs, aerobic exercise programs, and other means of habit control or behavior modification can be very helpful to the patient who is struggling to stop overeating, to stop smoking, and generally to get "back into shape."

The second issue to address is the pharmacological agents used for hypertension and their effects on sexuality and sexual functioning. These medications are frequently the same kinds of medications that are used in other types of heart disease.

CONCLUSION

Several different variables can affect the sexuality of the cardiovascular patient. Although there are many different levels of cardiac functioning, certain emotional responses seem to be present. Fear is the most common emotion. Therapeutic "talking" regarding fears and concerns is invaluable for patients who need to reconnect with their sexuality. Table 9-1 reviews some topics that can be covered.

Table 9–1
Guidelines for Cardiovascular Patients on Staying Sexually Active

1. The safety of sexual activity depends on your medical health. These guidelines are based on data such as medical history, general health, exercise testing, blood work, and electrocardiograms (EKG) and stress tests.

2. Join a cardiac rehabilitation program. A modifed aerobic health program can be helpful for your sex life because it can increase the efficiency of the heart. Aerobic exercise can increase cardiac reserve and therefore lower the stress on the heart during sexual activity.

3. Some medications for hypertension or cardiac disease can affect sexual functioning. If this occurs, it is important to notify your physician. Do not stop taking the medication! However, a dosage adjustment or medication change can often alleviate the problem.

4. When beginning sexual activity after a myocardial infarction, start slowly. Sometimes it is helpful to first use self-stimulation such as masturbation or nongenital activity such as massage, hugging, and kissing.

5. Try to avoid alcohol and heavy meals before sex.

6. Some sexual positions are more stressful than others in terms of creating dypsnea. Be creative and flexible in terms of "listening to your body." There is no inappropriate sexual position.

7. During sexual intercourse it is common for your heart rate to become faster or for you to breathe more heavily. However, you should not have chest pain. If this occurs, consult your physician. Frequently medication adjustments will help these symptoms.

8. Communication is essential to a healthy sex life. This includes communication with your partner, your nurse and your physician. Most problems can be successful handled through open, honest communication.

Chapter 10

Sex and Genitourinary Conditions

For almost two years now, Judy has tried to avoid sex with her husband. It wasn't that she didn't love him. At 57, after 30 years of marriage, she still cared deeply for him. It wasn't that she didn't like sex. She did. But the more sexually active they became the more likely she was to get another attack of cystitis. It felt miserable. She almost longed for those bygone days when she got her period. At least she didn't have all of those infections.

The following chapter will address sexuality issues related to genitourinary dysfunction. When reading this material it is important to consider the increased sense of body image discomfort and embarrassment the patient may be feeling, because the body systems involved within this group of diseases are related to the genitalia.

These patients also frequently experience multiple intrusive procedures to these organ systems. This may make them even more uncomfortable in addressing sexual concerns.

THE KIDNEY

Kidney disease can be very traumatizing in terms of dependency, life-threatening changes, and body image concerns. Chronic renal failure means that there is a decreased ability of the kidneys to maintain metabolic and fluid equilibrium in the body. The kidneys are not properly excreting excess salts and fluids that the body has ingested.

Frequently these patients need to go on dialysis to maintain a proper metabolic and chemical equilibrium. They are typically on many different medications and must also practice diet and fluid restriction. Dialysis frequently must be done three times a week, and patients must stay on the dialysis machine for approximately 4 hours. They are dependent on dialysis to stay alive.

There are many causes of renal disease. These include infections and congenital conditions such as polycystic kidneys. Chronic diseases such as severe hypertension, cancer, diabetes, and lupus may also affect the kidneys and cause them to stop functioning.

Physiological Responses

End-stage renal disease affects all parts of the body. For example, the skin may become itchy. The gastrointestinal tract may also be involved, and nausea and vomiting may occur with end-stage diabetes. Hypertension and cardiac problems may also exist, as well as anemia and neurological problems in the central and autonomic nervous system.

End-stage renal disease can alter mood. Depression is common and can be experienced as a sequel or possibly as the result of a chemical imbalance. Chronic fatigue due to all of the above physiological changes is also a common experience for the dialysis patient.

Infertility due to anovulation frequently occurs. Men may also become infertile because of impaired spermatogenesis.

As a result of all these conditions, all stages of the sexual response cycle can be affected. Examples of dysfunctions include erectile failures related to diabetic neuropathies and inhibited sexual desire as the result of fatigue and medications.

Body image distortions related to medication can be another side-effect. Patients on prednisone may develop what has been termed a "moon face." They may also experience large swings in their mood. Frequently they have steroid depression. Excess weight gain and fluid retention occur as a result of the kidney's inability to excrete salt and fluids properly. Finally, orgasmic problems related to the side-effects of medication and diabetic neuropathies are frequently present.

Psychosocial Responses

For the patient who is faced with chronic, progressive renal disease, the effects to sexuality may be devastating. Being dependent on dialysis, being unable to work, having multiple medical procedures, and having to limit food and water intake are part of the experience of this disease. Since dialysis also necessitates geographic dependence, vacations can be almost impossible. These are just some of the many issues that may affect body image, self-concept, and relationships.

Implications for Nursing

Assessment of sexual functioning should be included as part of the initial assessment. However, since sexual functioning may continue to change, it must be part of the ongoing nursing assessment.

Allowing patients and their partners to grieve and acknowledge the multiple losses that occur with this disease may be very helpful and may facilitate communication and intimacy. Helping couples negotiate concerns related to independence/dependence is also crucial. For example, maintaining comfortable sex roles is important for the emotional health of patients and their families. This may be difficult for patients who have to give up their job or dominant role as breadwinner. Nurses can make positive suggestions related to other roles and tasks the patient can help with in the family so that they can continue to feel purposeful and valued.

Patients who are transplant recipients may fare better and are frequently able to recover some of their sexual losses, including their fertility. Since pregnancy is not recommended for younger transplant patients for at least 2 years after transplant, they may need help regarding contraception options. Some transplant recipients also need permission to grieve for the donor patient and his or her family.

Organizations such as TRIO and KIDNEY-1 are important information sources for patients and their families. These groups are not only sources of information but also crucial links to the high-tech field of transplants. They are also important resources for emotional support.

BLADDER

There are several diseases that may affect the bladder. These diseases include bladder cancer and cystitis.

Cystitis

Cystitis occurs more frequently in women than in men because of the shorter length of the urethra (about 1 inch in the female). The proximity of the urethra to the vagina and rectum also makes the urethra more susceptible to ascending bacteria from these two body parts. Women who are postmenopausal are also at higher risk for acquiring these infections because of atrophic urinary tissue, which becomes depleted from lack of estrogen.

Older men are also more likely to develop cystitis. However, men typically develop cystitis as a result of a secondary mechanical problem such as an obstructed bladder neck. Contributing conditions include benign prostatic hypertrophy, prostate cancer, and bladder cancer, and bladder stones.

Cystitis is frequently treated successfully within 48 hours by antibiotics. However, the pain, frequency, and urinary burning can affect sexual desire.

Implications for Nursing

A sexual history is a very important assessment tool when working with the patient with this condition because frequently there is a relationship between sexual activity and cystitis. For example, women who have infrequent sexual activity and diminished vaginal lubrication are more likely to develop an infection after sexual intercourse than women who are routinely active sexually and have good vaginal lubrication.

The following care plan for the woman patient may be helpful in eliminating the frequency of cystitis.

1. Two to 3 quarts of fluid should be ingested daily to dilute the urine. To avoid excessive weight gain, drink nonsugary sodas. Acidify the urine by drinking cranberry juice and citrus juices.

2. Urinate every 3 to 4 hours. This will flush the urethra.

3. Wear cotton underpants and panty hose with a cotton crotch. This will help keep the perineum dry.

4. After defecation or voiding clean the perineum away from the vagina to the rectum.

5. Avoid bubble baths. They frequently are irritating.

6. Use unscented toilet paper.

7. Pat the perineum or use a hairdryer on the cool setting to dry it.

8. Avoid the use of a diaphragm for contraception. Diaphragms increase the possibility of developing a bladder infection.

9. Consider using a low-dose antibiotic as a preventative. This can be prescribed by your doctor.

10. Void before intercourse.

11. If postmenopausal, consider using estrogen cream or a water- soluble lubricant.

THE PROSTATE

The prostate gland is an important organ of the male reproductive system. It is a small, walnut-sized gland that basically wraps itself around the urethra just below the bladder outlet. The function of the prostate is to enhance semen by adding important nutrients and fructose to the seminal fluid. This provides an ideal transport medium which allows the sperm (produced by the testicles) to swim freely in search of an egg.

The various nutrients produced by the prostate help the sperm remain healthy and fertile.

Prostatitis

The prostate is a common site for infections. Symptoms of prostatitis include perineal and lower back pain. Urinary frequency and urgency are also common symptoms.

It is very important for the nurse to realize that although prostatitis can be treated with antibiotics, it tends to be "resistant" to treatment. This is because the prostate gland is like a sponge with many thousands of tiny secretory glands. Often medication does not reach all these glands.

Chronic prostatitis can cause lack of desire. It may also precipitate uncomfortable painful contractions during orgasm. Frequently men with prostatitis begin to avoid sex to prevent the pain of intercourse.

Implication for Nursing

The following nursing interventions may be helpful for the patient with chronic prostatitis.

1. Give factual and understandable information regarding the etiology of the problem.

2. Explain the importance of compliance during antibiotic treatment. Frequently patients discontinue their treatment prematurely if they are feeling better. Emphasize that they must complete a full course of antibiotic therapy.

3. Explain that they must drink a minimum of 2 liters of water a day unless contraindicated by their physician.

4. Direct them to use warm sitz baths and a mild analgesia for discomfort.

5. Suggest voiding before intercourse.

Benign Prostatic Hypertrophy

It is documented that a part of the normal aging process, beginning with middle age, is enlargement of the prostate gland. In fact, almost 50% of men 50 years and older and 75% of men over the age of 75 have an enlarged prostate.

Symptoms of *benign prostatic hypertrophy (BPH)* include "strangling" of the bladder outlet, which causes straining to void, urinary frequency, dribbling, urgency and excessive nocturia. The surgical complications of correcting the condition are well known, and many men fear and avoid the surgery. These complications include *retrograde ejaculation*, a medical condition in which the ejaculatory fluid is not expelled from the urethra but empties back through the bladder neck into the bladder. This condition causes functional infertility because the sperm are not excreted into the vagina. Erectile dysfunction may be another side-effect of the surgery if the nerves that affect erection are severed. However with advancing surgical techniques men are not experiencing as many postoperative sexual difficulties. However, these problems are still prevalent, and many men have heard the "war stories" of their peers.

A new promising medical therapy for BPH is Proscar. This drug can "shrink" the prostate gland and thus alleviate the "strangling" of the bladder outlet. Urinary flow is improved and surgery can be avoided totally for many men, or delayed 5 to 15 years for many other men.

Implications for Nursing

Nurses can give preoperative information regarding the possibility of retrograde ejaculation. Explaining how the bladder neck can be damaged during surgery demystifies this problem. It is important to include the partner during this conversation.

Addressing the couple's concern regarding erectile dysfunction is also helpful. Patients can unintentionally set themselves up for psychogenic impotence; that is, they will have erectile problems because the expect them, even if there is no physical cause.

Since this group of men is frequently older, we need to be sensitive regarding our own age and how this may contribute to a patient's and/or his spouse's discomfort. It is also very important to include the spouse in any conversations because frequently couples are uncomfortable talking about sexuality. If anxiety intrudes, the patient may not correctly process the information. Having another pair of "ears" is helpful for this reason as well.

Chapter 11

Sex and the Patient with Respiratory Disease

When he was a young man he had been a runner. That was before all of the cigarette smoking had caught up with him. Now, he could just barely go up the steps without having to stop once or twice on the landing. Sex. He just didn't have the energy. His wife said that it was "okay." They were too old anyway. But sometimes he just wanted to be able to do it again. If only he wasn't so short of breath.

Chronic obstructive pulmonary disease (COPD) is a collective term that refers to a group of respiratory diseases characterized by shortness of breath (dyspnea), easy fatigability, wheezing, and a productive cough.

One disease that produces these symptoms is asthma. Asthma is characterized by increased responsiveness in the patient's airway to certain environmental stimuli or "triggers" such as pollen, dust, and mold. Strong emotions and even exercise can precipitate an asthma attack. This increased sensitivity may result in bronchoconstriction, bronchospasm, and mucus hypersecretion.

Chronic bronchitis is another common respiratory condition. It is usually related to prolonged exposure to irritants. Although there are many occupational irritants, one common one is cigarette smoking. Symptoms include increased mucus secretion and cough.

Emphysema is also characterized by changes of the alveolar walls and progressive enlargement of the air spaces within the lung. Air becomes trapped and patients do not get enough oxygen. Usually patients who have emphysema also suffer from bouts of bronchitis.

This group of diseases can be very frightening for patients and their families. That is because many patients feel they cannot breathe. Other patients have increased dyspnea and fatigue. Frequently these patients may need portable oxygen.

PHYSIOLOGICAL RESPONSES

Since the average age of the COPD population is from 40 to 70 years, many of the normal changes related to aging are also beginning to affect sexual functioning. It is therefore important to give patients accurate information regarding what may be related to normal changes due to the aging process and what may be related to physical changes due to COPD. Frequently patients make inaccurate assumptions regarding their sexual functioning on the basis of myths and misperceptions.

A common physiological change seen in COPD include an increased incidence of arteriosclerosis. When the iliac arteries to the pelvis are clogged, Leriche's syndrome and impotence will occur. It is important to diagnose this syndrome because it is the only cause of impotence that can be corrected by surgery (by an aortic iliac femoral bypass). Another physiological change is a slowing of peripheral sensory and motor conduction, which may affect erectile functioning for males and orgasmic functioning for both males and females.

Severe hypoxia may make sexual activity difficult or even impossible because it has been determined that the energy needed for intercourse is equivalent to briskly walking two flights of stairs. Many chronic lung disease patients do not have that energy capacity.

Certain drugs used for COPD may also influence sexual functioning. These include the following:

1. Inhaled bronchodilators such as Proventil/Ventolin, Allupent, and Maxair. Because these drugs relieve shortness of breath, they can actually improve sexual functioning when they are used in proper doses. With proper dosage patients may also experience increased exercise tolerance.

    However, large overdoses of these drugs can impair sexual functioning by causing stimulation, tremors, and anxiety. The oral bronchodilators such as Theodur/Slo-Bid, Brethine, and Ventolin/Proventil can also have the same positive and negative effects on sexuality. Oral agents can occasionally cause severe nightmares.

2. Steroids, which are widely used for asthma, may cause infertility and menstrual irregularities. Mood swings both "up" and "down" are also a common experience: many patients become either euphoric (the short-term "high") or very depressed. Sometimes both occur. That is euphoria is followed by severe depression ("steroid crash"). Unless recognized, these steroid depression mood swings may affect a couple's relationship and family life in extremely negative ways.

3. Diuretics are widely used for COPD with secondary heart failure (cor pulmonale), may have positive effects on sexuality because they produce diuresis and therefore relieve congestive heart failure, which will enable more comfortable breathing. However, diuretics occasionally cause erectile dysfunction. Diuretics should also not be used within an hour or two of sexual activity as this may interfere because the patient may have urinary urgency.

4. Nicotine patches used to stop smoking are very useful in helping patients stop smoking. However, they too, may occasionally cause nightmares, which can influence sexual functioning.

EMOTIONAL RESPONSES

COPD may affect self-concept in a very negative way. Because of the debilitating nature of the disease, patients frequently are unable to work. Thus they may suffer from financial as well as personal loss in terms of work and family identity. Frequently patients and their significant others begin to feel anger and hopelessness. As the disease progresses, many patients experience a sense of separation from the world. Other patients may have a very difficult time with increased dependence on others. All of these stresses lower the desire for intimacy.

A patient's sense of body image can also become very negative. With increasing COPD, physical changes begin to occur. These include a "barrel" chest, distended neck veins, and "blue" cyanosis coloring of the skin. For individuals who value their physical powers, these changes in form and function may considerably alter their self-concept. Increased mucus production and cough may make it very unpleasant to engage in sexual activity.

All of the above experiences can contribute to depression and anxiety. Needless to say, these mood states can also negatively affect sexual desire and intimacy.

IMPLICATIONS FOR NURSING

The following interventions can serve as a guide in helping the patient who has COPD to maintain sexual functioning.

1. Education: Patients need to know that they should no longer smoke. Patients and their spouses need to understand the normal aging process and limitations specifically related to COPD. Encourage patients to participate in a pulmonary rehabilitation program.

2. Increase optimum factors when having sex: The following considerations may be helpful.

Time of day: What time of day does the patient have the most energy?

Environmental control: The room should not be too hot or cold. The "ideal" temperature is approximately 68° F with 40% humidity.

Diaphragmatic breathing: Exhaling through pursed lips for several minutes before sexual activity increases oxygen saturation.

Medication: Using a bronchodilator or inhaling oxygen (if not contraindicated) before sex can be helpful.

Positioning: The healthy partner can have a more active role. Two helpful positions include the side-lying position and the position with the male seated and then straddled. Pillows can be used to protect the chest. Some patients find that a waterbed is helpful because less movement is needed to have satisfying sexual intercourse.

Sexual activity should not occur after a heavy meal or alcohol consumption.

Emotions should be relaxed and tranquil.

Proper nutrition and rest should be maintained.

3.   **Sexual counseling:** Should include the following questions.

Discuss sexual assumptions and level of comfort. What is the belief system regarding sexual functioning? How comfortable is the couple with change? How do they feel about aging?

What was prior sexual functioning like for the couple?

What are the partner's issues? Is he or she healthy?

Also it is important to:

Encourage communication. Encourage the patient and family to participate in a support group.

The above suggestions are guidelines that can be used for both patient and family members. Respiratory diseases can be a challenge to sexual functioning. However, as noted, there are many important interventions that the nurse can make to help create a more positive sexual experience.

Chapter 12

Sex and the Patient with Diabetes

Nick had been diabetic since he was 16. Now, at the age of 50, he was not able to get an erection. In fact, for the past 7 years, sexual intercourse had become a difficult thing for him. He had just come from a lecture given by the local hospital where they discussed penile prosthesis. He wondered how his wife might feel about it. He had an appointment with the nurse diabetic educator next week. Maybe he should take his wife Ruth with him to the appointment and talk about this problem. . .finally. After all, Ruth had also been struggling with living with his diabetes.

Diabetes is a very common chronic disease. It is believed to be caused by either a lack of insulin secretion from the pancreas or decreased uptake of glucose by the muscles in the body. Without appropriate levels of insulin, the glucose needed for carbohydrate metabolism is not available.

Although diabetes is an endocrine disorder, both a vascular and a neurological component contribute to its pathology and disability. Both of these components also affect sexual functioning.

There are several symptoms that are commonly experienced when diabetes is "out of control." These include polyuria, polydipsia, fatigue, pruritus, and visual changes. Although diabetes can occur anytime during the life cycle, it commonly occurs as *juvenile-onset diabetes*, which almost always requires insulin for treatment (insulin-dependent diabetes) and *adult-onset diabetes*, which usually does not require insulin for treatment (non-insulin-dependent diabetes). Adult-onset diabetes most commonly occurs during the sixth and seventh decade of life. It is also more common in obese men and women and often can be controlled.

There are several ways that diabetes can affect sexual functioning. Because the issues are different for each gender, the following discussion will address these differences.

THE DIABETIC MALE

Erectile dysfunction is occasionally the presenting symptom that will alert the patient or the physician that the patient may have diabetes. Patients will have problems achieving and maintaining an erection. This dysfunction may develop over a period of several months or even years. The changes that are responsible for the erectile dysfunctions are believed to be a combination of neurological damage and vascular insufficiency rather than endocrine problems related just to the high blood sugar.

Studies have shown that peripheral neuropathies seem to be the cause of erectile dysfunction in approximately 30 to 60% of men. Neuropathies may cause an inability to maintain an erection. However, decreased blood flow due to circulatory problems influences penile circulation and may also interfere with maintaining an erection.

Diabetes seems to have very little effect on other parts of the sexual response cycle. For example, the desire and orgasmic phases of the cycle seem to be unchanged. However, retrograde ejaculation does occur more frequently in diabetic men and is believed to be caused by a pelvic autonomic neuropathy. This neuropathy inhibits the reflex closure of the sphincter of the bladder neck after emission and before expulsion of semen. Rather than going through the penis, semen flows back through the relaxed bladder spincter and into the bladder.

Fertility can also be influenced, again because of retrograde ejaculation. There may also be an increase of abnormal sperm production.

THE DIABETIC FEMALE

In terms of sexual functioning, the excitement phase of the sexual response cycle seems to be most affected in diabetic women. Women seem to have more vaginal dryness. This may be caused by the high level of glucose in the blood. Increased blood sugar can contribute to yeast infections as well.

Another problem for the diabetic woman is related to a possible elevated stimulatory threshold before orgasm. This means that it may take increased amounts of stimulation for the woman to reach orgasm. This can be a very uncomfortable feeling. It may also be exhausting for both the patient and her partner. The female diabetic may also have problems related to reproduction. Pregnancy may severely tax the pancreas and cause difficulty in regulating insulin. However, with today's better monitoring devices for blood glucose levels, more diabetic women are able to not only conceive but also have healthy babies.

IMPLICATIONS FOR NURSING

There are several nursing considerations which are applicable for the diabetic patient. In addition to those listed below, see Table 12-1.

1. Education: This includes education to prevent complications. Encourage the patient to lose weight if they are overweight and stop smoking. Discuss the importance of keeping blood pressure under control as well as increasing one's exercise (with the physician's collaboration).

2. Keeping blood sugars under control will help patients stay healthy with good sexual functioning and will thus prevent further problems. Make sure patients are on a healthy diet and encourage them to stay on that diet.

3. Infertility in males may be addressed via artificial insemination.

4. Impotence: Although we do not want to encourage psychogenic impotence (meaning that the mind is creating the problem), patients should be knowledgeable about the disease process. If impotence develops, look for treatable causes first, for example, blood sugar that is out of control, drug side-effects, Leriche's syndrome, and depression. There are several kinds of penile prostheses available that will help the male maintain an erection if erectile problems develop. This may be a sensitive subject for either the male or his partner; however, these prostheses may be very effective in enhancing sexual functioning. Many are inconspicuous.

5. Female diabetics should be careful to avoid yeast infections. Preventive measures include wearing cotton underpants, staying only in dry bathing suits, eating the proper foods, and avoiding stress.

6. Couples may frequently need sexual counseling to address their concerns. This should be an ongoing process.

Table 12–1
Guidelines on Maintaining Sexuality for Diabetes Patients

1. Approximately 50% of diabetic men will experience some form of sexual problem at some time during their illness. The most frequent sexual problem is low sexual desire in both men and women and erectile problems in men. Education and open-ended communication are crucial.

2. Diabetic women are not at higher risk for sexual problems than healthy women. However, they are at higher risk for decreased

vaginal lubrication. A water-based soluble lubricant can be very helpful in maintaining lubrication.

3. Couples need to be aware that diabetes is not the only reason for a dysfunction. Frequently, problems are caused by both relationship issues and the stress of a chronic disease.

4. The physical changes that occur as we age in the sexual response cycle become accelerated with a male who has diabetes. For example, diabetic men may find that they need more sexual stimulation to have an erection and as discussed diabetic women may need more stimulation to have an orgasm. This is important for couples to understand. Many spouses believe that this is the result of lack of interest in the partner, when actually it is a side-effect of the disease.

5. Semen production may eventually decrease as the diabetes progresses. It is important to consider this physiological change if fertility is going to be important, especially for younger couples who do not have any children. At this time, we have sperm banks to freeze sperm for future use. These issues should be discussed before a problem occurs.

6. Couples need time to talk and process their feelings. If necessary, they should set aside a time of the day or week to focus on their concerns.

7. Sexuality does not have to end in intercourse to be pleasurable. Encourage couples to enjoy the process of lovemaking. It is also important not to place unrealistic demands on a partner.

8. Other health problems and health habits can have a negative influence on sexuality. These include any of the chronic diseases and also habits such as cigarette smoking and alcohol.

9. Patients should keep in regular contact with their physician and nurse, who can be invaluable sources of information. Remind them that it is important to ask for help or information.

Chapter 13

Sex and the Patient with Cancer

Judy looked at her ring. Only 3 more weeks until her wedding. Imagine a bride with no hair! Phil had been really kind. He had told her that it wasn't her hair that he had fallen in love with. It was her. Still, she was glad that she had bought that beautiful wig. No one had to know that she had lost her hair with the last round of chemotherapy. Chemotherapy was difficult. But at least she would look good for the wedding.

PHYSIOLOGY OF CANCER

The term *cancer* is derived from *karkinos*, the Greek word for crab. Throughout history, cancer has been a much feared and dreaded disease. In fact, cancer can be considered to be many different diseases with similar characteristics.

Prior to the 20th century cancer was perceived as a death sentence for the patient. Only in very recent history have we openly discussed with cancer patients their diagnosis and treatment. The mortality rate from cancer has greatly improved in the past 30 years: 50% of newly diagnosed patients with cancer can now be expected to live 5 years. Survival rate has been greatly enhanced by high-tech medical treatments such as linear accelerators and sophisticated chemotherapy and new chemotherapy agents.

In terms of pathology, cancer is characterized by uncontrolled local proliferation of cells, with invasion of adjacent normal structure. Distant spread is called metastasis. This usually occurs through either the bloodstream, through the lymphatics, or within a body cavity.

About 1 million new cases of invasive cancer appear each year and half that number die every year. Cancer is ranked second behind heart disease as a leading cause of death in the United States. The mortality rate has declined for the population that is less than 65 years of age. Cancer is frequently experienced as a disease of the elderly.

PSYCHOLOGICAL REACTIONS TO CANCER

The societal reaction to cancer is slowly becoming less stigmatizing. However, the special problems associated with cancer, such as pain, disfiguring tumors, concerns about contagion, loss of attractiveness due to surgery, radiation, or chemotherapy still create huge psychosocial problems. Studies have shown that approximately 50% of all cancer patients are depressed or highly anxious. One result of this altered mood state is that sexuality and intimacy may be severely challenged as patients lose their sexual desire.

It must be remembered that each neoplasm has it own idiosyncratic features by virtue of its location, treatment approach, and severity. All attempts to enhance sexual functioning must therefore address the unique characteristics of each kind of cancer.

Nurses should also be aware of the myths regarding cancer in our society. These myths or belief systems frequently hinder our ability to make positive interventions for the patient. They include the following:

Cancer is catching.

Cancer equals death or pain.

Once the air hits it. . .

Cancer equals poverty.

Cancer is everywhere.

Cancer is shameful.

SEXUAL COMPLICATIONS OF TREATMENT

The most common sexual dysfunctions related to cancer treatment in men are erectile dysfunctions, impotence, retrograde ejaculation, infertility, loss of libido or desire, and loss of sex organs via "surgical castration."

In women, the most common sexual dysfunctions related to treatment include loss of a breast and stenosis and atrophy of the vagina. Menstrual irregularities and infertility are other common problems. Some women experience early menopause as a result of surgical castration. These may cause body image distortion, dysparunia and lack of desire.

Both men and women often lose interest in sex during cancer treatment. Initially, this lack of desire is linked to concern for survival. However, treatment may contribute to continued loss of desire because of the anxiety, depression, and physical side effects that frequently accompany radiation, chemotherapy, or surgery.

Nausea related to chemotherapy and/or pain related to the cancer or the treatment can also interfere with sexual desire. Many of the chemotherapy agents also interfere with normal hormonal balances. Hormone therapy, which is frequently given for prostate cancer and breast cancer, may affect the desire phase in both men and women and cause erectile dysfunctions as well as breast enlargement (gynecomastia) in men.

Cancer treatment frequently interferes with all parts of the sexual cycle. For example, it can interfere with erection by upsetting the male's hormonal balance or by damaging his pelvic nerves (demyelination). Orgasms may become painful (this may be experienced by some women as well). Premature ejaculation or painful ejaculation in some men may also occur. Cancer surgery, including radical prostatectomy and radical cystectomy, can also influence ejaculation and erectile function.

Abdominoperineal resection and pelvic exenteration surgery for colon cancer may affect all phases of the male sexual response. Similarly, radical hysterectomy and pelvic exenteration for cervical, uterine, and ovarian cancers, as well as radical cystectomy, may affect all phases of the sexual response cycle for women.

Radiation can affect the sexual response cycle by making intercourse painful and can also contribute to infertility. In the younger woman radiation to the pelvic area may cause the ovaries to stop secreting estrogen. If the radiation dose is large enough this will cause infertility or precipitate menopause if the radiation can destroy ovaries so they cannot heal and recover.

Pelvic radiation may also cause inflammation and distress; examples of these conditions are radiation cystitis, radiation colitis, and radiation proctitis in adjacent organs. As healing occurs, scar tissues (adhesions and strictures) may form. These effects tend to be dose related. Vaginal stretching through intercourse or the use of a vaginal dilator can help prevent scarring.

Approximately a third of the men who receive radiation notice a change in the quality of their erections. Radiation therapy affects erection by damaging the arteries (sclerosis) that carry blood to the penis and by damaging the nerves (demyelination) that stimulate the penis. These effects are also frequently dose related. Testosterone production may also slow down with radiation. In men, as in women, scar tissue can form, resulting in adhesions and strictures.

IMPLICATIONS FOR NURSING

Nursing interventions need to address both psychological and physiological complications. They include emotional support, accurate information regarding what to expect from the cancer, and education and counseling regarding sexuality.

The American Cancer Society has two excellent patient information publications on cancer and sexuality, one for the male and one for the female. Both publications are comprehensive and well written and will be a helpful aid to nursing interventions. They are called *Sexuality and Cancer; For the Man Who Has Cancer and His Partner, and Sexuality and Cancer; For the Woman Who has Cancer and Her Partner*. These books are useful guides for any medical professional who is working with sexuality concerns.

When educating the patient who has cancer, nurses should cover the following topics:

1. Information about the sexual response cycle and how cancer may affect its functioning

2. Enhancing sexual interest

3. Coping with body image changes such as hair loss, weight gain or loss, and surgical losses; the Look Good—Feel Better Program sponsored by the American Cancer Society has been developed to help men and women cope with body image changes via the use of make-up and wig.

4. Discussing risks for developing infertility and appropriate options, including sperm and egg banking before infertility becomes permanent.

5. Depression and anxiety and techniques to cope with these feelings such as counseling, relaxation techniques, guided imaging and music and human therapy

6. Specific interventions to prevent sexual problems and to cope with sexual pain

7. Coping with multiple losses and their influence on self-esteem

8. Communication and intimacy skills for couples

9. Resources available for more intensive family, couple, and sexual counseling

10. Support groups

Part IV

Sexual Problems and Positive Interventions

This part of the book reviews some of the key concepts related to sexual functioning. The three chapters that follow address specific areas that are important for the nurse to understand. Many of the topics presented are usually not discussed within a nursing curriculum and therefore are not typically within the nurse's knowledge base. Hopefully, this overview will give you further insight into the complex study of human sexuality.

Chapter 14

The Sexual Anatomy and the Sexual Response Cycle

THE SEXUAL ANATOMY

It is important to be aware of the anatomical structures that constitute the male and female reproductive tracts. The following is a brief discussion of the sexual anatomy of the male and female.

The female sexual anatomy includes the following body parts (see Figure 14-1):

The external genitals	The internal genitals
Labia majora	Hymen
Labia minora	Greater vestibular glands
Clitoris	Vagina
Mons pubis	Cervix
Urethra	Uterus
	Fallopian tubes
	Ovaries
	Bladder

FIGURE 14–1
Female Reproductive Organs

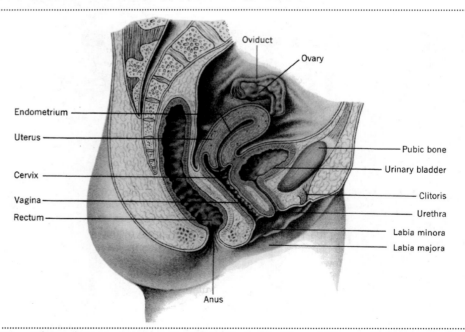

From Burke, *Human Anatomy & Physiology in Health and Disease*, 3rd ed., Delmar Publishers, 1992.

The male sexual anatomy includes the following body parts (see Figure 14-2):

The external genitals	**The internal genitals**
Penis	Testes
Scrotum	Epididymis
Urethral meatus	Vas deferens
	Seminal vesicles
	Prostate gland
	Ejaculatory ducts
	Bulbourethral glands
	Bladder

FIGURE 14-2
Male Reproductive Organs

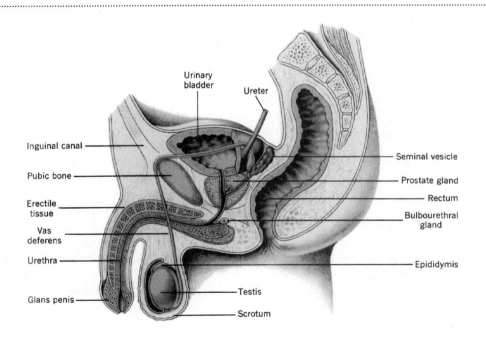

In both males and females, the brain and the skin are also considered to be sexual organs.

From Burke, *Human Anatomy & Physiology in Health and Disease*, 3rd ed., Delmar Publishers, 1992.

THE SEXUAL RESPONSE CYCLE

The sexual response cycle is a wonderful example of the interconnectiveness of all the dimensions that affect sexual expression. The focus of the following material will be on the physiological and anatomical aspects of sexuality so that you can give patients accurate information regarding normal sexual expression. Sexual dysfunctions, or "problems," are discussed in the following chapter.

A four-phase model of human sexual response was first described by Albert Moss in 1909 and by Wilheim Reich in 1942. Then in 1966 Masters and Johnson observed over 10,000 episodes of sexual activity in 382 women and 312 men in a laboratory setting. From their observations they determined that the sexual response cycle was composed of four stages: excitement, plateau, orgasm, and resolution. These stages are not strictly delineated and may vary not only in different people but with the same person during different sexual experiences.

Masters and Johnson believe that there are two basic physiologic reactions during the human sexual response. The first is *vasocongestion*, which causes an increased amount of blood to concentrate in the genitals. In females there is also an increased concentration of blood in the breasts. The second physiological reaction is increased neuromuscular tension, or *myotonia*. Myotonia occurs throughout the body in response to sexual arousal.

Helen Singer Kaplan (1977), a prominent sex researcher, added anothermore dimension to this cycle: desire. She believed that desire was the catalyst for the sexual response cycle. Her model, called the triphasic model, includes the desire state, the excitement phase, and the orgasm phase.

Another very interesting interpretation of the Sexual Response Cycle was presented by David Reed (1984), who correlated the sexual response cycle with a more psychological response. He outlined the following four phases:

Seduction: corresponds to the desire phase

Sensation: corresponds to the excitement phase

Surrender: corresponds to the orgasm phase

Serenity: corresponds to the resolution phase.

For a diagram of these various models, see Figure 14-3.

FIGURE 14–3
Model of the Sexual Response Cycle

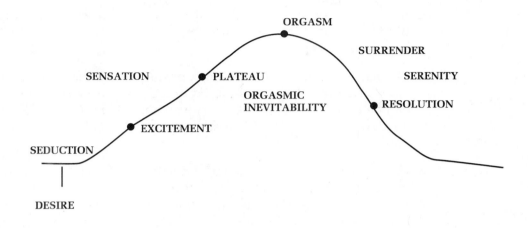

This author believes that the sexual response cycle is composed of Kaplan's stage of desire and Masters and Johnson's four stages.

- *Desire* is influenced by many different factors. These include environmental stimuli, cultural factors, health, past experiences, and physiology. There is also a very strong psychological component to this stage. Desire is the precursor to the initiation of the sexual response cycle and "sets the stage" for the individual to be receptive to sexual stimuli. Desire is motivation or interest in sex.

  In terms of physiological stimulation, desire probably depends on certain hormones such as androgen, testosterone, and possibly the neurotransmitter dopamine, all of which increase sexual desire. High levels of the pituitary hormone prolactin may suppress sexual interest and pleasure. Current data also suggest that women's sexual desire peaks just before and after the menstrual cycle.

- *Excitement:* Excitement is felt through the body via physiological and psychic stimuli. There is also a subjective component to this stage because the ability to focus on pleasurable genital sensations is related to permission giving and comfort. With adequate stimulation, either by tactile or psychogenic (emotional) stimuli, intensity increases; with withdrawal of stimuli excitement disappears.

Sexual excitement is easier to measure physiologically than desire because men and women show signs of generalized arousal similar to that observed with other strong emotions.

- In the *plateau* stage sexual tension becomes intensified to the point of orgasmic inevitability. Muscle tension is now independent of emotional stimuli.

- *Orgasm* is an involuntary climax or release of increased sexual tension through strong muscular contractions. Although the total body can be involved, the most intense area is the genitalia. Like desire and excitement, this stage also has physiological and psychological components.

- In *resolution*, physical changes bring the body back to the preexcitement state. Females can be restimulated at this point, whereas males have a period of time known as the *refractory period* before sexual excitement can begin to increase again. This period of time becomes longer as men age.

For detailed summaries of physiological changes in this cycle, see Tables 14-1 and 14-2.

Table 14-1
Physiological Changes That Occur for the Male During the Sexual Response Cycle

Excitement phase

1. The penis becomes erect.

2. The scrotal sac thickens and flattens; the scrotum elevates.

3. The testicles elevate and slowly increase in size.

4. In some men there is nipple erection.

Plateau phase

1. The penile coronal circumference increases.

2. The testicles increase by as much as 100%.

3. The testicles continue to elevate.

4. Sex flush may be present in about 25% of men.

5. Carpopedal spasm occurs.

6. Increased muscular tension, respirations, blood pressure, and pulse occur.

7. Small amount of secretion from Bulbourethral gland (this is called emission) occurs.

Orgasmic phase

1. Ejaculation: this may also occur before orgasm.

2. Contraction of the accessory organs. These include the vas deferens, seminal vesicles, and ejaculatory duct.

3. Relaxation of the external bladder sphincter and concurrent contraction of internal bladder sphincter.

4. Contractions in the penile urethra: 0.8-second intervals for up to 3 or 4 contractions.

5. Anal sphincter contractions.

6. Continued increase in blood pressure, respirations, pulse, and muscle tension.

Resolution phase

1. There is a rapid loss of pelvic congestion.

2. Erection is lost. This occurs during a two-stage process: an initial 50% loss, and then a gradual loss of the rest of the erection.

3. There may be an increase in sweating in a small percentage of men.

4. Decrease in tachycardia, blood pressure, and muscle tension.

5. Increased feelings of fatigue and need to rest.

Table 14-2
Physiological Changes That Occur for the Female During the Sexual Response Cycle

Excitement phase

1. Vaginal lubrication (approximately from 10 to 30 seconds).

2. The vaginal walls and labia thicken.

3. The inner two-thirds of the vagina expands.

4. The corpus uterus and the cervix elevate.

5. The clitoris becomes enlarged.

6. The nipples become enlarged.

7. A sex flush may occur in some women.

Plateau phase

1. There is full expansion of the vagina to allow the penis to enter.

2. The outer one-third of the vagina reaches its orgasmic platform.

3. The uterus and the cervix elevate.

4. There is a mucoid secretion.

5. The clitoris retracts to be completely covered by the clitoral hood, and its length decreases by about 50%.

6. A sex flush occurs in about 75% of women.

7. Increased muscle tension, respirations, blood pressure, hyperventilation, and tachycardia.

Orgasmic phase

1. The uterus contracts from the area of the fundus to the lower uterine segment.

2. There may be mild relaxation of the external cervical os.

3. Contractions of orgasmic platform: 0.8-second intervals for 5 to 12 contractions.

4. The external rectal sphincter contracts as well as the urethral sphincter.

5. Hyperventilation, tachycardia, and increased blood pressure.

Resolution phase

1. Some women are rapidly able to return to orgasm without loss of pelvic vasocongestion.

2. Rapid loss of flush in labia minora and orgasmic platform.

3. Clitoris loses tumescence.

4. Sweating in about 30 to 40% of all women.

5. Hyperventilation may still persist.

6. Decrease in tachycardia, blood pressure, and pulse.

7. Sense of relaxation.

It is interesting to note that there are many similarities between the male and female sexual response cycle in terms of physiological changes. The major difference between men and women seems to be that about 13% of women can experience multiple orgasms, whereas men enter a refractory period soon after orgasm. The later orgasms for women typically require less stimulation than the initial orgasm. Female orgasm generally also has more variability than male orgasm.

The Sexual Disorders

This chapter addresses the types of sexual problems that a patient may experience. The nurse should be familiar with normal sexual functioning as discussed in the prior chapter.

Two major categories of sexual disorders are deviations and dysfunctions. The deviations are not caused by chronic or acute medical illness but may be related to psychological trauma or mental illness.

SEXUAL DEVIATIONS

> His name was Mark, but he believed and wished that he could be called Mary. From his earliest memories he always felt as if his mind was trapped in the wrong body. His parents, especially his father, just couldn't understand how he felt. They took him from psychiatrist to psychiatrist to help him "get better."
>
> As he got older and was able to move away from home he, slowly began to change his body with hormones. If only he didn't feel trapped in this male body. If only he could be a woman.

Although the arousal stimulus in people with deviations differs from the accepted norm, sexual deviations are characterized by good and pleasurable sexual functioning. This is not true with sexual dysfunctions (discussed below), which typically do not involve pleasurable and satisfying sensations. For example, men with deviations may achieve good erections and women may be sexually arousable.

It has been theorized that sexual deviations develop as the result of traumatic events that occurred during the early part of childhood. As a result of these experiences, the child's mind creates erotic associations that are not within the normal range of such associations.

John Money labeled the beginning of these associations "vandalized lovemaps." He believed that the most vulnerable age for nonerotic behavior to be perceived as sexually stimulating was between the ages of 6 and 9. As nurses we therefore need to be aware of the vulnerability of these young children and try to avoid intrusive procedures whenever possible.

Sexual deviations may respond to a variety of therapeutic interventions, such as insight and behavioral and pharmacological agents. However, they are not responsive to standard sex therapy techniques.

Among behaviors that would fall into this category are *gender identity disorders* such as *transsexualism*, typified by the scenario at the beginning of this chapter. In this disorder patients feels that they are trapped in the wrong gender body. They have a sense of discomfort and inappropriateness about their anatomic sex and frequently wish to be rid of their own genitals. These patients frequently ask to undergo sex-change surgery so that their physical bodies will be more congruent with their psychological status.

The majority of sexual deviations include the *paraphilias*, frequently called by the lay public "perversions." Paraphilias feel sexually aroused by specific inanimate objects or activities. Without these objects or activities they are unable to be sexual or "turned on." Some of the paraphilias are culturally defined: they may be considered abnormal by our culture and historical era. For example in certain agricultural societies sex with animals, such as sheep is considered to be an acceptable sexual act and is even encouraged as a sexual release, whereas in many other cultures this is considered to be a paraphilia and even punished by death.

The paraphilias include *fetishisms*, or the use of nonliving objects for arousal, and *transvestism*, the use of cross-dressing for the relief of tension or gender discomfort. Other paraphilias include *zoophilia*, or sexual experimentation with animals; *pedophilia*, or sexual acts with children; and *exhibitionism*, or repetitive acts of exposing the genitals to an unsuspecting stranger for the purpose of achieving sexual excitement with no attempt at further sexual activity with the stranger. *Voyeurism* (peeping Tom), *sexual masochism* (violent or painful sexual acts against oneself), and *sexual sadism* (violent or painful sex acts against another) are other paraphilias.

Of all the paraphilias, pedophilia is probably one of the most common and disturbing because children are involved. This involvement can alter the child's life in many negative ways. Pedophilia is also one of the most common causes of multiple intrapsychic trauma in children, adolescents, and adults.

Many of the patients that the author has counseled over the years have been victims of sexual abuse as children. These patients are typically women. The intrapsychic damage is frequently reflected in lack of desire, sexual aversion, sexual promiscuity, and in extreme situations multiple personality disorders (MPD). How women react to this experience is colored by a myriad of factors that include the age when they were abused, the relationship of the abuser to the woman, the nature and frequency of the abuse, and the reactions of other family members to this frequent family "secret." In all states nurses are legally obligated to report suspicious sexual abuse of children.

SEXUAL DYSFUNCTIONS

> For the past year every time that he tried to make love he found he would get more and more anxious. His wife would get angrier and angrier. Lately, he just tried to avoid sex. He would watch television until he thought that she might be sleeping. He just couldn't understand why he could no longer keep an erection. He felt terrible and his wife felt rejected.

Sexual dysfunctions are the most common way to describe a sexual problem. Although there are no definitive figures on the prevalence of sexual difficulties in the general population, research on specific populations has shown that serious sexual dysfunctions exist in 9 to 63% of relationships.

We need to be aware that sexual dysfunctions may be culturally and socially defined. What may be seen as sexually appropriate and acceptable behavior in one culture or situation may be viewed as a dysfunction in another. For example, in some cultures it is not acceptable for women to have orgasm. Therefore anorgasmia would not be defined as a problem in those cultures. In other situations it may feel advantageous for the male to reach orgasm quickly. In those situations, therefore, the male would not be considered to have a problem with premature ejaculation.

We also need to be aware of assessing or labeling the potential for sexual problems within the context of the couple. If the couple has the same level of desire, there typically is not a problem. It is when partners have different sexual needs that concerns about dysfunctions may occur. For example, if one member of the couple wants to have sex twice a day and the other member wants to have sex twice a week, there could well be a "sexual problem" that needs intervention.

The sexual dysfunctions are based on the first three phases of the sexual response cycle: desire, excitement, and orgasm. They can also be global or situational. *Global dysfunctions* occur in every sexual encounter. Dysfunctions can also be viewed as primary or secondary. *Primary dysfunctions* typically suggests a lifelong problem, whereas *secondary dysfunctions* usually suggest a problem that has developed after a period of satisfactory sexual functioning.

Desire Phase

Disorders of desire include *inhibited sexual desire*, which is becoming increasingly common. This can be defined as persistent and pervasive inhibition of sexual desire. For desire to be present, the patient must feel and be interested in feeling sexual and must be attentive to sexual stimuli.

Sexual aversion, which is much more rare, can also occur. Men or women who experience sexual aversion find that all aspects of sexuality repulse them. Sexual aversion is usually felt to be psychogenic in origin.

Causes of problems within the desire phase include hormonal problems such as a low testosterone level or elevated prolactin level, depression, alcohol, conflicts and issues concerning intimacy, fear of loss of control, negative messages from parents and the culture, childhood sexual abuse and trauma, and myths regarding sexuality. One such myth is that sex is always supposed to be spontaneous.

Although the Diagnostic and Statistical Manual of Mental Disorders (DSM-IIIR) does not include a category for excessive sexual interest, *sexual addiction*, is now being perceived as a problem for some patients. These patients use sex like alcohol or drugs, as a means of coping with their lives. When they are unable to be sexual, their discomfort level becomes unbearable.

Excitement Phase

During the excitement phase both subjective experiences and absence of physiological arousal can cause dysfunctions. Among the many disorders within this group are: decreased subjective arousal, difficulty in achieving an erection, and difficulty in maintaining an erection.

Erectile dysfunctions can also be primary or secondary. It is not uncommon for men complaining of erectile dysfunctions to obtain full erections upon awakening or through masturbation despite their inability during sexual activity with a partner. The most common disorder related to erectile dysfunction is known as *impotence*, which can be defined as the inability to obtain or maintain erections sufficient for penetration 25% or more of the time.

Some of the major causes of this group of disorders are anxiety and depression. Physiological problems related to vascular and neurologic deficits can also cause erectile dysfunctions. Both a psychological and medical work-up are necessary in this area of dysfunction.

Some of the questions related to the medical work-up for the male would include whether the erectile problem was gradual or sudden, the presence or absence of morning erections, the affect of the person (depressed, etc.), and whether or not erection is achieved by masturbation. Questions related to the medical work-up of the female would include the presence or lack of vaginal lubrication, control issues in the relationship, and fantasies and thoughts that are pleasurable or fearful. Other problems for women include vaginal tightness and dryness.

For women, a problem that can occur during the excitement phase is *vaginismus*, a painful involuntary spasm of the pubococcygeal muscle upon penetration or thrusting by the penis. Vaginismus is almost always a phobic response and is frequently seen in women who have been raped or sexually abused as children.

Dyspareunia, or painful intercourse, can also occur in some women and less commonly in men. This condition always warrants a medical examination. This should include a careful history of the nature and timing of the pain, scarring or anatomical problems, and vaginitis. Hormonal insufficiency resulting in vaginal atrophy, as well as endometriosis, or pathology of the uterus, the broad ligaments, or the fallopian tubes, may also contribute to the problem in women.

Many diseases can influence the excitement phase.

Systemic diseases such as chronic obstructive pulmonary disease, chronic renal failure, angina or congestive heart failure, neurological degenerative disorders, malignancies, and infections

Endocrine disorders such as hypothyroidism, Addison's disease, hypopituitarism, acromegaly, diabetes, and Cushing's disease

Conditions related to testicular functioning such as bilateral orchitis due to mumps, TB, trauma

Vulva and vaginal pathology: imperforate hymen, infection

Damage to androgen supply from oophorectomy plus adrenalectomy

Orgasmic Phase

The essential pathology related to orgasmic dysfunction is the involuntary inhibition of the orgasmic reflex. Orgasm may be affected in many different ways. For instance, some men and women may have *anorgasmia*: they are not be able to have an orgasm at all.

There is also a considerable amount of anxiety and emotionality related to this phase of the sexual response cycle because of the mythology related to the appropriate way that an orgasm should occur. This is especially true for women. Many men and women believe that an orgasm should originate from the vagina. However, for women it is the clitoris that is usually essential in orgasm. In reality there are several kinds of orgasms in women. They include both the vaginal and clitoral orgasm. The cultural orgasm typically results from stimulation of the clitoris during masturbation as well as coitus whereas vaginal orgasms are thought to be the result of direct stimulation of the vaginal wall.

Some men may have orgasm too quickly, a condition called *premature ejaculation*. Such men have lost voluntary control over the ejaculatory reflex. It takes 7 to 10 minutes of thrusting for men to achieve orgasm; however, that time varies from man to man and from situation to situation.

Other men and women have difficulty in achieving an orgasm. This condition is called *inhibited orgasm* in women or *retarded ejaculation in men*. *Ejaculatory incompetence* is an orgasmic condition in which the male cannot ejaculate into the vagina. This is almost always psychogenic in origin.

The quality of the orgasm can also be of concern. Some men ejaculate with no sensation of pleasure. This condition is called *anhedonic orgasm*. A more common condition is orgasm with lessened pleasurable sensations.

Another common problem for men is that of "dry" orgasm, during which there is no ejaculation. This is seen frequently in diabetic men and also following prostate surgery. In this *retrograde ejaculation* the ejaculate goes into the bladder rather than out through the penis.

Various diseases can cause these sexual problems during the orgasmic phase.

Systemic disease which affects both erection and ejaculation. They include pulmonary disease, renal disease, cardiovascular disease, degenerative diseases, malignancies and infections

Endocrine disorders such as hypothyroidism, Addison's disease, hypopituitarism, acromegaly, feminizing tumors, Cushing's disease, Klinefelter's syndrome, and diabetes

Local genital disease: priapism, chordee, Peyronie's disease, penile trauma, balanitis, phimosis, herpes, lower back pain, urethritis, prostatitis

Mechanical problems that may affect performance: chordee, hypospadias, hydrocele, hernias, penile injury, priapism, mutilation or absence.

Damage to genitals and their nerve supply by prostatectomy, abdominal or perineal bowel resections, abdominal aortic surgery

Castration

Neurological disorders: malnutrition and vitamin deficiency, spina bifida, surgery or trauma to the lumbar, sacral or spinal cord, pelvic parasympathetic nerve plexus injuries, multiple sclerosis, pelvic radiation "burns," and injury

Vascular diseases that impair erection: leukemia, trauma, sickle-cell disorders, hyper-coagulation disorders

Local pathology in women: clitoral adhesions, tight clitoral hood, pubococcygeal muscle weakness or fibrosis

It is not important for nurses to memorize and recognize the etiology of every sexual dysfunction. What is important is to recognize when a dysfunction does exist and help the patient contact the appropriate resource person.

Sexual History Taking, Counseling, and Sex Therapy

This chapter discusses the PLISSIT model of intervention, sexual history taking, and techniques of sex therapy. The intent is not to encourage you to become sex therapists, but to enable you to be more comfortable regarding the various techniques used by counselors and sex therapists so that you can be more helpful to your patients and their families. Another goal of this chapter is to enable you to become more comfortable with your own boundaries and become aware of when it is appropriate to consult a therapist.

THE PLISSIT MODEL OF INTERVENTION

About 75 to 80% of sexual counseling and education can be appropriately done by the nurse or someone who has some background in sexuality issues. The PLISSIT model is a guideline for helping you assess when it may be necessary to seek more experienced professionals.

P = Permission Giving: Frequently by just introducing the topic of sexuality we give patients permission to begin to discuss a topic or ask a question that they may have. Talking about sexuality may also give them permission to engage in certain sexual activities.

LI = Limited Information: Many patients need simple, basic information regarding their illness or have questions regarding normal life development issues.

SS = Specific Suggestions: Some patients need more specific suggestions. For example, patients who are having pain with intercourse because of arthritis may need help in finding a comfortable position.

All of the above interventions may be within the scope of nursing practice.

IT = Intensive Therapy: Examples of people needing intensive therapy might include women and men who have been sexually abused and have lost their sexual desire and men who have erectile dysfunction as the result of diabetes and marital conflict. These issues need not only nursing interventions but also supportive and psychotherapeutic interventions.

Use this guideline to address your own qualifications and limitations and to give yourself permission to seek additional resources when necessary.

THE SEXUAL HISTORY

The sexual history is an important part of patient care because both the emotional and physical health of patients can be affected by their sexual health. The various components of the history are interconnected. For example, conflicts in sexuality can result in depression, anxiety, alcoholism, and obesity. Obesity can then lead to diabetes and hypertension, and hypertension can lead to impotence. This circularity can manifest itself in numerous other examples.

Taking a sexual history demands greater skill than taking any other health history because questions regarding sexuality can elicit many anxiety-ridden emotions, as well as embarrassment, discomfort, and even anger. Thus the interviewer needs to be aware of not only technical questions but also of the affective responses that may occur.

Ideally, a sex history should be taken when the initial full medical or nursing history is taken. Including this part of the assessment during the initial stage of information gathering communicates to patients that sexuality is an integral part of health care and that the health professional is comfortable addressing these questions and concerns. Omission of these questions may be a loud statement of discomfort.

Frequently "secrets" are not shared during this initial phase. Perhaps at a later date these important components of the sexual history can be approached again. But this early demonstration of comfort with this subject and permission to talk about sexual concerns may later prove to be invaluable.

Guidelines for Taking a Sexual History

Several guidelines can be used to create a comprehensive and successful sexual history that enables patients to be more comfortable and therefore more honest in voicing their concerns to you. A good sexual history also correctly assesses and incorporates age-appropriate questions.

1. Each interviewer should use an opening statement that feels comfortable and that will begin to develop a therapeutic relationship. For example, the opening statement can include the following:

   Since I am going to be working with you as your nurse during your hospital stay, it is very important that I am aware of what your needs will be. One important area that I would like to address with you today is that of your sexual health. Unfortunately, in the past this area was usually ignored, but we are now beginning to understand how important sexual health may be to your mental and physical well-being.

Therefore, I am going to ask you several questions related to sexuality that in my experience seem to be very relevant for beginning to plan for your care. They will include questions regarding sexual functioning, perhaps some of the types of sexual experiences you have had, sexual preferences, how satisfying your marital intimacy has been, and any questions you might have regarding how your illness may be affecting your sexuality. You need to know that what we discuss is medically confidential and that if you have any discomfort in answering my questions you should let me know.

2. Interview the patient in a quiet, private, relaxed environment. Although this is not always possible, it is much more difficult to begin to talk about sensitive subjects when other people are in the room. Privacy acknowledges respect for the individual.

3. Acknowledge, affirm, and normalize feelings and behaviors. It is okay to acknowledge that the questions may be sensitive and may trigger uncomfortable feelings. It is important for the patient to understand that discomfort is not a negative behavior and that such feelings occur frequently when we address issues that are usually ignored.

4. Gather the educational material that you need to be able to help guide patients. Be prepared to answer questions. You should have a working base of knowledge so that you can begin to give patients accurate information. Know what your resources are and how you can access them.

5. Practice good interviewing strategies:

- Begin the interview with the least sensitive questions. For example, questions about marital status or dating beliefs are probably less threatening to answer than questions related to masturbation or sexual orientation. As trust and comfort begin to develop, you should be able to ask more sensitive questions. Emotionally charged questions should be approached gradually.

- Move from the general to the more specific. Begin with questions regarding the presence of intimacy rather than the "mechanics" of intimacy.

- Ask questions beginning with "when?" and "how often?" rather than "do you?" These are called "ubiquity" questions because topics are introduced with the assumption that most people have experienced what is going to be asked. From these questions you may become more specific with "what has been your experience?"

- Introduce a question using the third person. An example of this style would be "Some people find that when they have diabetes they may have problems with erection."

- Move the question from the past to the present. Usually questions related to past history are more comfortable and easier to address than concerns that are in the present.

- Questions should progress from learning to attitudes to behavior. The nurse can ask what a patient has learned about a certain behavior before asking how the patient feels about the behavior or if the patient has ever acted upon the actual behavior.

6. Use appropriate language geared to the patient. It is sometimes difficult to have the patient understand what you are saying and not sounding offensive by using street language. Be sure your language is age appropriate. Children and very anxious patients may need more explanation and simpler terminology.

7. Be aware of very sensitive topics. These may include teenage or childhood sexuality, sexual abuse, sexual dysfunctions, masturbation, affairs, abortion, date rape, and sexual assaults.

8. Adjust your interview style and questions to be age appropriate. The following are general guidelines of what may be age-related or developmental concerns.

- **Childhood:** Most sexual interviewing of young children takes place in front of their parents. Often we are placed in the role of educator and are attempting to correct myths and misperceptions for both the parent and the child.

  Frequently the normalcy of childhood sexual behavior is an issue. Parents may be as anxious as the child. Communication with the very small child is usually more successful through the use of toys such as action figures, anatomically correct dolls, and coloring.

  What we are trying to also understand are family attitudes about emotional expressiveness, physical affection, and sexuality. Other considerations are the parent's ability to help the child have a sense of autonomy and self esteem. The child's sense of body image is another aspect to consider as well as childhood experiences of sex play and masturbation.

Children who have been sexually abused or have had other very negative sexual experiences may also have a great amount of discomfort or even acting-out behavior such as irritability, excessive silliness, or crying and clinging to their parents.

- **Adolescence:** Since confidentiality is frequently an issue for the adolescent, the interviewer must be very aware of the ethics and rules of confidentiality and be "up front" with the teenager. Although they may act differently than they feel, most adolescents are very embarrassed to talk to an adult about sexual concerns. These concerns frequently include teenage pregnancy, contraception, sexual orientation, and fears regarding intimacy, and STDs. Concerns regarding changing body image and appropriate sexual behavior may also worry the adolescent.

- **Early adulthood:** Young adulthood is a time of increasing separation from parents and establishing intimacy with others. Comfort regarding sexual orientation may be an important issue. Other concerns may include performance anxiety, anxieties about new relationships, pregnancy, birth control options, abortion, and miscarriage.

- **Early midlife (30–40):** At this stage many couples are coping with marital and intimacy issues. Infertility may also become an issue if they have waited to the end of this stage to become pregnant. Past experiences with trust, loss, and change of sexual partners may also be a concern. Privacy issues are frequently a concern because this age group may have small children and also teenagers.

Later midlife (40–60): In the early part of this stage couples are frequently questioning their relationship. The physical process of aging becomes obvious as well as the occurrence of chronic disease. Menopause and sexual changes related to aging also occur. Frequently men and women may seek sex with others to pretend that they are still young. Some women may experience an increase in sexual desire after menopause when they no longer have to worry about birth control and becoming pregnant.

- **Later life (after age 60):** Anxieties related to diminished sexual functioning can be of concern, as well as depression, chronic disease, and multiple losses. Nurses need to be very aware of the myths related to aging because the patient may frequently believe them. They include the belief that sex is only for the young and is not appropriate for the elderly. Aging plays a role in a person's self-image, sexual functioning, and sexual activity.

9. Give the patient the opportunity to ask for a referral. Frequently, when the patient begins to share important or sensitive information, it becomes apparent that further sexual counseling might be appropriate. Let the patient be aware of the resources that may be helpful. This would include trained therapists as well as support groups and reading materials.

The above components are guidelines to enable you to create a sexual history that is comprehensive, relevant, and sensitive to the needs of the patient.

A Model of a Sexual History

The following sexual history illustrates a comprehensive interview for the patient with chronic disease. The questions included cover some of the issues that you might want to address. This is a generic guideline and should be adapted to fit the setting and the needs of the clinician and patient.

Sexual History for the Chronic Disease Patient

1. Physical factors

    General health: What has been the quality of your health prior to this time?

    Concurrent illness: Do you have any other health problems?

    Previous surgeries: Have you had any prior surgery? At what age? How has this surgery interfered with your sexuality?

    Medications: What medications do you routinely take? What medications do you take only when needed? Have you noticed any possible effects of your medications on sexual functioning?

    Energy level: Are you feeling fatigued? What time of the day is the "best" time for you in terms of being and feeling energetic?

Symptoms of illness: What symptoms are you experiencing presently? Are they having an impact on your life?

Side-effects of treatment: What kinds of treatment are you getting? Are you experiencing any side-effects such as fatigue, nausea, vomiting, or diarrhea?

Body image changes: How has this illness changed how you perceive your body? Are you able to adjust to these changes? Have you shared these feelings with your significant other? If you are not in a relationship, has this influenced you in any negative way?

Health of partner: Does your partner have health issues? How do these problems affect his or her sexuality? How do they interfere with your sexual functioning? Have these problems been discussed?

2. Psychological factors

Depressive symptoms: Do you feel life is worth living? Have you noticed a change in your mood? How are you sleeping? Too much, too little, just enough? Do you have problems falling asleep? Do you have early morning awakening? How is your appetite? Are you enjoying your life?

Anxiety: How do you typically handle anxiety-producing situations? Have you noticed any physical signs such as your heart beating fast, sweating, or feeling too hot or too cold? Are you able to concentrate?

Prior and present coping behaviors: In the past, when you have had a difficult situation, what coping strategies have you used to help you work through the problem? Have they been successful?

Prior history of psychiatric or emotional problems: Do you have a history of depression or anxiety? Have you ever been hospitalized for a psychiatric or emotional problem? Have you ever been given medication for an emotional disease?

Life-situational stressors: What else is going on in your life at this time? How is your family? Do you work? Have you had any major achievements or disappointments in the past year? Any major changes in your life?

Loss: Have you lost anyone close to you in the past year? Who or what have you lost in recent times that could influence the way that you might be feeling?

Religious orientation: Is religion an important part of your life? Do you consider yourself religious? Do you ever seek out your religious leader?

3. Relationship factors

Marital status: What is your marital status?

Duration of relationship: If you are in a relationship, how long has this been? Have you just left a relationship?

Number and ages of children: How many children do you have, and how old are they? Are you responsible for any children from any prior relationships? How are the children doing?

Prior quality of relationship: Before this illness, how would you describe the quality of your relationship or marriage? How well are you able to communicate with one another? Can you usually count on one another when there are problems?

Definition of sex roles: How do you believe that men and women should behave? What has been your role in the relationship? Has it changed since the illness? How do you see it changing in the future? What concerns do you have regarding these changes?

Strengths and weaknesses of the relationship: How do you see the relationship? What concerns do you have regarding the relationship now that you may be having sexual problems? What positive coping skills have you as a couple used in the past? How easy or difficult is it for you to share your concerns?

Importance of intimacy within the marriage: What is the role of intimacy within your marriage? Are you able to communicate your needs?

4. Sexual factors

These questions are very important for taking a helpful sexual history.

Desire present or absent: Do you desire sex? Has this desire increased or decreased since your illness?

Prior sexual drive and interest: Have you noticed any problems in your ability to have and enjoy sexual relations?

Orgasm: Do you have any problems having an orgasm?

Repertoire of sexual behaviors: Are you able to use all of your five senses during sex? Is there any sense that is a problem for you, for example, seeing, tasting, or smelling?

Use of fantasy: Do you use fantasy? Are you comfortable with it? If not, what messages did you learn about fantasy?

Interest and health of partner: Is your partner interested in having sex? Are there any limitations for him or her?

For the male:

Erections: Do you have any problems having an erection? Do you have morning erections? Can you maintain an erection with masturbation?

Orgasm: Do you have any problems having an orgasm? Do you ejaculate (come) too soon or not soon enough? In what situations do you have these problems?

For the female:

Dyspareunia: Does intercourse hurt? If it does, under what circumstances? Do you have problems with lubrication?

Vaginismus: Do you have problems when you try to have genital intercourse? Are you experiencing painful spasms when attempting intercourse? Can penetration occur?

If there is a sexual problem, ask the patient the following clarification questions:

How much of a problem is this for you and your partner?

What goes on in your mind when you try to have sex?

How do you and your partner react to the problem?

How long has this been a problem?

Do you have any ideas about what causes the problem?

5. Nursing Assessment and planning should also take the following factors into consideration:

Myth and beliefs about illness and sexuality: What have patients heard regarding what happens to their sexuality from their illness? Have any of their friends or family had this disease? What have they shared with the patient? Some people believe that . . . (fill in what you believe is appropriate to help you get an idea of their belief system).

Cognitive level: What is the developmental level of the patient?

Feelings about genital organs: What were and are the messages and the feelings that they have regarding their genitals?

Perception of current illness: How do they view this disease? Are they optimistic? Do they feel guilt or shame?

Flexibility: How willing do they seem to cope, make adaptations, and test new behaviors? Do they seem rigid in their belief system? Who are they willing to allow into their world to help them adapt?

Previous sex education/counseling/therapy: What has been their past experience with many of the above modalities? Has it been positive or negative? Why did they seek out the information or the counseling?

SEX THERAPY

It is not typically in the scope of nursing practice to do sex therapy. However, it is important and interesting to understand some of the basic techniques that are included in this form of therapy.

Originally sex therapy was usually planned as short-term therapy which lasted approximately 10 to 20 sessions. It was symptom oriented and based on behavioral techniques: this means that the couple or the individual was given specific tasks to practice to help overcome the problem.

Masters and Johnson devised various sensate-focus exercises to help people become comfortable with their own ability to get aroused. This technique uses progressive desensitization to help overcome sexual problems and to gain trust and confidence. Couples are given "home-work" assignments that help them become more comfortable with their sexuality or to help control "problems" such as inhibited desire or lack of desire, impotence, and orgasmic dysfunction in the female. The techniques used in this therapy are frequently useful in not only helping patients overcome their sexual problems but also in increasing communication and intimacy.

The following three examples of sensate-focus exercises illustrate the typical sequence and methods used to help patients overcome their sexual problems. They are typically planned to occur over several weeks or months. Because couples are often uncomfortable, frequently these exercises are introduced by education videos and during counseling sessions.

Sensate-Focus Exercise 1: Inhibited Sexual Desire

1. Basic equipment might include a large bath towel and a bottle of oil or lotion. Oil is better in the winter because it has a warming effect. Lotion is usually more comfortable in the summer because it is more cooling. Tell them to keep the lights on and find a comfortable spot.

2. Emphasize that excitement and orgasm cannot be willed by either partner.

3. Instruct the couple to massage each other without touching the genitals. Tell them to try to become more aware of their genital sensations as they are being stroked. Tell them to listen to the feelings of their partner's fingers as the partner gently caresses their body. Have them concentrate on what they are feeling and continue to keep their body relaxed.

4. Encourage communication regarding pleasurable sensations.

5. Tell the couple to take turns lying on their stomach and fully relaxing their body. They should alternately tighten and relax their muscles, from their head down to their toes. They should practice tightening and relaxing their body. If they can, they should close their eyes and imagine that they are floating.

6. Have them turn over so that the stroking can be repeated on the rest of their body. Throughout the activity they can describe out loud what feels pleasurable.

7. Tell them to slowly start genital stimulation. This may not occur for several weeks or months. Do not have intercourse yet. Repeat the exercise several times, emphasizing what is most pleasurable. If the

partner wishes to have orgasm, tell them they can help the partner achieve orgasm by caressing the partner's body.

8. Have them change places.

Sensate-Focus Exercise 2: Orgasmic Dysfunction in the Female

1. Emphasize that orgasm cannot be willed, nor is it a requirement every time the couple has intercourse.

2. Emphasize that orgasmic response in the female is a matter of accepting various pleasurable and erotic physical stimuli.

3. Emphasize that the female must communicate with the male, stating what is most stimulating and pleasurable for her.

4. Emphasize that sensitivity among both partners is most crucial at this stage.

5. Instruct the couple to begin to slowly initiate genital stimulation with the female sitting and straddling the male's legs with her back against the male's chest.

6. She begins by squeezing his legs, holding his hands, and guiding his hands in a stroking or caressing manner, however feels best for her.

7. During this early stage the male may caress, massage or stroke all parts of the female body except the clitoris.

8. Communication and sensitivity continue, emphasizing sensual desire rather than forced responsitivity.

9. A "teasing" approach may be tried by the male as he stimulates, strokes, massages, and caresses both the sexual and nonsexual parts of the female body.

10. When vaginal lubrication increases, the clitoris may be gently stimulated by manual stroking.

11. When the female becomes excited, intercourse can be initiated with the female in the top position.

12. Vaginal containment of the penis is a goal at this stage.

13. The couple continues to communicate what is most pleasurable for the female, and she becomes comfortable in her ability to communicate what gives her pleasure.

14. The male then may begin slow, nondemanding thrusting of the penis.

15. Intercourse may be stopped, and the couple may start all over again with gentle caressing and lovemaking.

16. Intercourse is then repeated in different positions, first in the lateral position, then with the male on top.

17. Communication always continues in a nondemanding and nonjudgmental manner.

18. Pleasure and trust are emphasized, not mandatory orgasm by the female.

19. Orgasm should occur naturally as the female develops confidence and trust.

Sensate-Focus Exercise 3: Impotence

1. Emphasize that no man can will an erection.

2. Emphasize that anxiety has a potent inhibiting effect on sexual pleasures.

3. Deemphasize performance.

4. The female begins by gently stroking the partner's nongenital areas: arms, legs, neck, and back.

5. The male should communicate with the partner regarding what are pleasurable feelings.

6. The female begins to gently stroke the partner's genitals.

7. The male continues to communicate with the partner as to what feels best.

8. The female stimulates the partner until an erection occurs. Do not have intercourse.

9. Let the erection subside.

10. Repeat the stimulation again until the partner has another erection. Do not have intercourse.

11. Let the erection subside.

12. Repeat the stimulation again until the partner has an erection and begins to gain confidence in his ability to achieve and maintain an erection.

13. Let the female assume the top position and slowly have the penis enter the vagina.

14. Emphasize vaginal containment of the penis, then being slow thrusting backward and forward by the female.

15. Then let the male begin slow thrusting of the penis.

16. Communication continues, emphasizing sensate pleasure and vaginal containment.

17. Never emphasize climax, orgasm, or performance.

18. Gradually the couple will interact sexually in a very gratifying and pleasurable manner.

Marital Therapy

It is now obvious that frequently sex therapy needs to be done in conjunction with marital therapy. It has been estimated that as many as 75% of couples coming for marital therapy also have sexual problems. It is also believed that 50% of couples have sexual problems at some time. Many therapists have concluded that frequently sex therapy needs to be combined with marital therapy to be successful. Typically marital therapy includes insight-oriented therapy that looks at not only the present events but also the past history that couples bring into the relationship. Together, these two forms of therapy can be helpful in enhancing the quality of intimacy for the couple.

Conclusion

Sexual counseling and sex therapy are important assessment and intervention tools that can enhance the quality of life of your patients and their significant others. The interconnection of the mind and the body is powerful, and sexual functioning can only be enhanced when this connection is respected.

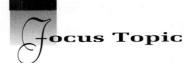

Focus Topic

Reading List for Patients and Professionals

Bibliotherapy is a powerful technique for enhancing sexuality because reading helps increase knowledge and may also create a sense of normalcy and comfort with sexual concerns. The following is a brief overview of some of the books that are available.

Sexuality

Masters, W. H., Johnson, V. E. & Kolodny, R. C. *Masters and Johnson on sex and human loving.* Boston, MA: Little, Brown, 1986.

Fun for Couples

McCarthy, B. & McCarthy, E. *Sexual awareness: Enhancing sexual pleasure.* New York: Carroll and Graf, 1984.

O'Connor, D. *How to make love to the same person for the rest of your life (and still love it).* Garden City, NY: Doubleday, 1985.

About Men

Kaplan, H.S. *How to overcome premature ejaculation.* New York: Brunner/Mazel, 1989.

Keen, S. *Fire in the belly: On being a man.* New York: Bantam, 1991.

Zilbergeld, B. *The new male sexuality.* New York: Bantam, 1992.

About Women

Barbach, L. *For yourself.* New York: Signet, 1975.

Barbach, L. *For each other.* New York: Signet, 1982.

Britton, B. *The love muscle: Every woman's guide to intensifying sexual pleasure.* New York: New American Library, 1982.

Boston Women's Health Book Collective. *Our bodies ourselves.* New York: Simon and Schuster, 1976.

Autoerotic Guides

Dodson, B. *Sex for one: The joy of masturbation.* New York: Harmony, 1987.

Gay Sex

Marcus, E. *The male couple's guide to living together.* New York: Harper and Row, 1988.

Silverstein, C., & Picanco, F. *The new joy of gay sex.* New York: Harper Collins, 1992.

Relationships

Hendrix, H. *Getting the love you want: A guide for couples.* New York: Harper and Row, 1988.

Sager, C.J., & Hunt, B., *Intimate Partners.* New York: McGraw Hill, 1979.

Scarf, Maggie. *Intimate partners: Patterns in love and marriage.* New York: Ballantine Books, 1987.

Sexual Abuse

Davis, L. *Allies in healing: When the person you love was sexually abused as a child.* New York: Harper-Perennial, 1991.

Davis, L. *The courage to heal workbook.* New York: Harper and Row,1990.

Graber, Ken. *Ghosts in the bedroom: A guide for partners of incest survivors.* Deerfield Beach, Florida: Health Communications, 1991.

Sexuality

Fogel, C. *Sexual health promotion.* Philadelphia: Saunders, 1990.

Green, R. (Ed.). *Human sexuality: A health practitioner's text.* Baltimore: Williams and Wilkens, 1979.

Kaplan, H. S., *Illustrated manual of sex therapy,* New York: Quadrangle: 1975.

Kaplan, H. S. *Disorders of sexual desire and other new concepts and techniques in sex therapy.* New York: Brunner/Mazel, 1979.

Lieblum, S., & Rosen, R. (Eds.). *Principles and practice of sex therapy; update for the 1990s.* New York: Guilford Press, 1989.

Lopiccolo, J., & Lopiccolo, L. (Eds.). *Handbook of sex therapy.* New York: Plenum, 1978.

Masters, W. H., & Johnson, V. E. *Human sexual response.*
Boston: Little,Brown, 1966

Masters, W. H., & Johnson, V. E. *Human sexuality* (4th Ed.). Harper Collins, 1992.

McDaniel, S. *Medical family therapy: A biopsychosocial approach to families with health problems.* New York: Harper Collins, 1992.

Money, J. Lovemaps: *Clinical concepts of sexual/erotic health and pathology, paraphilia, and gender transpositions: In childhood, adolescence and maturity.* New York: Irvington Press, 1986.

Schover, L., R., & Jensen, S. B. *Sexuality and chronic illness: A comprehensive approach.* New York: Guilford, 1988.

Schoever, L. *Sexuality and cancer: For the man who has cancer and his partner and sexuality and cancer: For the woman who has cancer and her partner.* American Cancer Society, 1988.

Relationships

Coutois, C. *Healing the incest wound: adult survivors in therapy.* New York: Norton, 1988.

Gurman, A.S., & Kristem, D. P., *Handbook of family therapy.* New York: Brunner/Mazel, 1991.

Martin, P., *A marital therapy manual.* New York: Brunner/Mazel, 1976.

Weeks, G., & Treat, G.S. *Couples in treatment: Techniques and approaches for effective practice.* Brunner/Mazel, 1992.

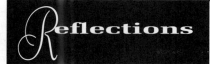

Reflections

On concluding this book, I find that I have many different thoughts and feelings on the subject of sexuality and more specifically our patients' sexuality. The most poignant one is related to the importance of our role as nurses in enabling our patients to hold on to their sexuality throughout the life cycle and still cope positively with the challenges that are constantly occurring throughout their lives.

It has been my experience that sometimes the smallest, simplest intervention can create the difference between losing one's sexuality and expression and keeping this great gift. I think frequently about one such example of how we can help a patient stay connected to his sexuality.

Arthur was a 39-year-old man with a very aggressive brain tumor. On the day of his discharge from the hospital, one of the nurses overheard Arthur and his wife talking. They were talking about where Arthur should sleep when he got home. This surprised the nurse because she had viewed them as a loving and caring couple. Why would they be discussing where Arthur should sleep?

Her curiosity became very strong, and she admitted to Arthur and his wife that she had overheard them talking and was confused as to why they were discussing sleeping arrangements. His wife answered that she loved Arthur very much and couldn't bear to sleep next to him and not be sexual. He felt the same way about her. They thought that they were no longer allowed to have sex because it might hurt him. *There was no reason why Arthur could not be sexual, but no one had told him that he was allowed to have sex if he wanted to, and he was too embarrassed to ask his doctor or nurses.*

The nurse called me. For the next hour or so Arthur, his wife, and I spoke about intimacy and the need to be held. We spoke about the possibility that Arthur might not be able to get an erection and that sex would be forever different for them. They grieved together for their potential losses as a couple, but, they also celebrated the fact that they could be sexual. They could hold one another, kiss one another, pleasure one another, and sleep in the same bed.

All this happened because as nurses we gave this couple the permission to talk and ask about their sexual concerns. Arthur went home knowing that he didn't have too long to live. But he also went home knowing that for whatever time he had left, sexuality did not have to be another one of his losses.

This simple intervention gave this couple back their innate right to be sexual. That is what this book is about. If you can close it and remember just a few thoughts or feelings that you had as you were reading, maybe, when you too, meet someone like Arthur, you can also help him or her remain empowered and sexual. That's what nursing is all about—empowerment, caring, educating, connecting, and enabling patients to live as full and happy a life as possible.

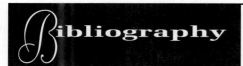 ibliography

Alexander, B., McGrew, M., & Shore, W. Adolescent sexuality issues in office practice. *American Family Practice*, October 1991, pp. 1273-1281.

Altherr, T. *Procreation or pleasure? Sexual attitudes in American history.* Malabar, FL: Robert Krieger, 1983.

Baker, R., & Elliston, F. (Eds.) *Philosophy and sex.* New York: Prometheus Books, 1984.

Barash, D. P. *Aging: An exploration.* Seattle, WA: University of Washington Press, 1983.

Barnett, R., & Baruch, G. Women in the middle years: A critique of research and theory. *Psychology of Women Quarterly*, 1978, 3(2), 187-197.

Bassili, J. On the dominance of the old-age stereotype. *Journal of Gerontology*, 1984, 36(6), 682-687.

Bogren, L. Changes in sexuality in women and men during pregnancy. *Archives of Sexual Behavior*, 1991, 20(1), 35-45.

Bruess, C., & Greenberg,J. *Sex education: Theory and practice.* Belmont, CA: Wadsworth, 1981.

Bullough, V. *Sexual Variance in Society and History.* New York: John Wiley & Sons. 1976.

Butler, R. N., & Lewis. M. I. *Midlife love life.* New York: Harper and Row, 1986.

Chodorow, N. Family structure and feminine personality. In M. Rosalo & L. Lamphere (Eds.) *Women, culture and society*, (pp. 43-66), Stanford, CA: Stanford University Press, 1974.

Cutler, W. B., & Garcia, C. R. Perimenopausal sexuality. *Archives of Sexual Behavior,* 1987, *16*, 225-234.

Erikson, E. H. *Identity and the life cycle.* Psychological issues. (Monograph 1). New York: International Universities Press, 1959.

Fisher, D. H. *Growing old in America.* New York: Oxford University Press, 1977.

Florence, M. E. A survey of sexual interest in an older adult population. *University Microfilms International.* (Unpublished presentation)

Freud, S. Some psychological consequences of the anatomical distinction between the sexes. In S. Freud, *The standard edition of the complete psychological works of Sigmund Freud* (vol. 19, pp. 253-260). James Strachey (trans.). London: The Hogarth Press, 1925.

Freud, S. Female sexuality. In S. Freud, *The standard edition of the complete psychological works of Sigmund Freud*. (vol. 21, pp. 223-243). James Strachey (trans.). London: The Hogarth Press.

Frieze, I., & Parson, J. *Women and sex roles*. New York: Norton, 1978.

Geltner, S. A historian's approach. In Kirkpatrick (Ed.) *Women's sexual development*. New York: Plenum Press, 1980.

Gilbert, H., & Roche, C. *A women's history of sex*. London: Pandora, 1988.

Gilligan, C. *In a different voice*. Cambridge, MA: Harvard University Press.

Goldman, A. The effects of a sex and aging workshop highlighting permission and limited information on the sexual knowledge, attitudes, behaviors and satisfaction of a group of older heterosexual couples experiencing erectile dysfunction: A quasi-experimental and qualitative design. U.M.I. Dissertation Information Service, 1991.

Green, R. *Human sexuality: A health practitioner's test*. Baltimore: William and Wilkins, 1980.

Haas, K., & Haas, A. *Understanding sexuality*. St. Louis, MO: Times Mirro/Mosby, 1987.

Holland, J. C., & Rowland, J. *Handbook of psychooncology: Psychological care of the patient with cancer*. New York: Oxford University Press, 1989.

Hyde, J. S. *Understanding human sexuality*. New York: McGraw-Hill, 1986.

Jones, R. E. *Human reproduction and sexual behavior*. Englewood Cliffs, NJ: Prentice-Hall, 1984.

Kaplan, H. S. *The new sex therapy: Active treatment of sexual dysfunctions*. New York: Times Books, 1974.

Kinsey, A.C., Pomeroy, W. B., Martin, C. E., & Gebhard, P. H. *Sexual behavior in the human male*. Philadelphia: Saunders, 1948.

Kinsey, A.C. *Sexual behavior in the human female*. Philadelphia: Saunders, 1953.

Klopovich, P. M., & Clancy, B. Sexuality and the adolescent with cancer. *Seminars in Oncology Nursing*, February 1985, pp. 42-48.

Lark, S. *The menopause self-help book*. Berkeley, CA: Celestial Arts, 1990.

Levinson, D. A conception of adult development. *American Psychologist*, 1986, *41*, 3-13.

Lewis, M. Female sexuality in the United States. In Kirkpatrick (Ed.), *Women's sexual development*. New York: Plenum Press, 1980.

Lewitte, H. Women's development in adulthood and old age: A review and critique. *International Journal of Mental Health*, 1982, *11*, 115-134.

Lief, H. (Ed.). *Sexual problems in medical practice*. Monroe, WI: American Medical Association, 1981.

LoPiccolo, J., & Miller, V. H. A program for enhancing the sexual relationship of normal couples. *The Counseling Psychologist*, 1975, *5*,(12), 67-72.

Ludeman, K. A review of the literature of sexuality and aging. T*he Gerontologist*, 1981, *21*(2), 204-207.

Lurie, H. J. *Clinical psychiatry for the primary care physician*. Nutley, NJ: Hoffman-LaRoche, 1976.

Mahler, M. S., Bergaman, A., & Pine, F. *The psychological birth of the human infant: Symbiosis and individuation*. New York: Basic Books, 1975.

Masters, W. M., Johnson, V. E., & Kolodny, R. C. *Human sexual response*. Boston: Little, Brown, 1966.

Masters, W. *Sex and human loving*. Boston: Little Brown, 1988.

Masters, W. *Human sexuality*. New York: Harper Collins, 1992.

Mazur, A. U. S. trends in feminine beauty and overadaptation. *Journal of Marriage and Family Counseling*, 1986, *22*(3), 281-303.

McDaniel, S., Hepworth, J., & Doherty, W. *Medical family therapy: A biopsychosocial approach to families with health problems*. New York: Harper Collins.

Morokoff, P. Sexuality in perimenopausal and postmenopausal women. *Psychology of Women Quarterly*, 1988, *12*, 489-511.

Munjack, D., & Oziel, J. *Sexual medicine and counseling in office practice*. Boston: Little, Brown, 1980.

Neugarten, B. L. Time, age and the life cycle. *American Journal of Psychiatry*, 1979, *136*(7), 887-894.

Notman, M. T. Women and Mid-life: A different perspective. *Psychiatric Opinion*, 1978, *15*(9), 15-25.

Oaks, W., Melchiode, G., & Ficher, I. (Ed.). *Sex and the life cycle: The thirty-fifth Hahnemann Symposium*. New York: Grunne and Stratton, 1976.

Olds, S. W. *The eternal garden: Seasons of our sexuality*. New York: Times Books, 1985.

Papalia, D. *Human development*. New York: McGraw-Hill, 1989.

Pfeiffer, E., Verwoerdt, A., & Wang, H. S. Sexual behavior in middle life. *American Journal of Psychiatry*, 1972, *128*, 1262-1267.

Pfeiffer, E., Verwoerdt, A., & Wang, H. S. Sexual behavior in aged men and women. *Archives of General Psychiatry*, 1968, *19*, 753-758.

Rossi, A. S. Life-span theories and women's lives. *Journal of Women in Culture and Society*, 1980,*6*(1), 4-32.

Rubin, L. *Women of a certain age*. New York: Harper Books, 1979.

Sarrel, L., & Sarrel, P. *Sexual turning points: The seven stages of adult sexuality*. New York: Macmillan, 1984.

Schover, L. R., & Jensen, S. B. *Sexuality and chronic illness: A comprehensive approach*. New York: Guilford Press, 1988.

Secunda, V. *By youth possesses: The denial of age in America*. New York, Bobbs-Merrill, 1984.

Selekman, J., & Simpson, G. Sex and sexuality for the adolescent with a chronic condition. *Pediatric Nursing*, November/December, 1992, *17*(6).

Shipes, E., & Lehr, S. Sexuality and the male cancer patient. *Cancer Nursing*, October 1982, pp. 375-381.

Simons, R. (Ed.). *Understanding human behavior in health and illness*.(3rd ed.). Baltimore: William and Wilkins, 1984.

Sontag, S. The double whammy of aging. *Saturday Review*, 1972, *55*(39), 29-38.

Starr, B. D., & Weiner, M. B. *The Starr-Weiner report on sex and sexuality in the mature years*. New York: McGraw Hill, 1981.

Tannahill, R. *Sex in history*. New York: Stein and Day, 1980.

Tarvis, C., & Sadd. *The Redbook report on female sexuality*. New York: Dell Press, 1977.

Wall-Hass, C., Nurses' attitudes toward sexuality in adolescent patients. *Pediatric nursing*, November/December 1992, *17*(6).

Wilson, J. *Women: Your body, your health: The essential guide for well-being*. New York: Harcourt Brace Jovanovich, 1991.

Wise, T. Sexual problems in cancer patients and their management. *Psychiatric Medicine*, 1985, *5*(4), pp. 329-341.

Woods, N. F. *Human sexuality in health and illness*. St. Louis, MO: C. V. Mosby, 1979.

Zawid, C. A descriptive study of female sexuality in midlife: Implications for the development of sex education. U.M.I. Dissertation Information Service. Unpublished Dissertation, 1990. (Unpublished Dissertation)

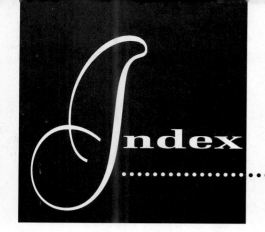

Index